DATE		

COOKING CREATIVELY FOR YOUR DIABETIC CHILD

COOKING CREATIVELY FOR YOUR DIABETIC CHILD

Caroline Hastings Babington

Foreword by Charles A. Carabello, M.D.
ILLUSTRATED BY MONA MARK

Doubleday & Company, Inc., Garden City, New York, 1979

ISBN: 0-385-14809-7
Library of Congress Catalog Card Number 78–20055

This book is dedicated to my daughter, Sherry, and to my husband, Ben. It was because of Sherry's diabetic condition that I first decided to undertake this task. It was Ben who gave me the support that I needed to complete my endeavor. He was my typist and my taster. He has been patient in his role and without him I might still be thinking about the book I would like to write.

FOREWORD

How fortunate to have a book written by a well-qualified dietician directed to diabetic children! Mrs. Babington's book will undoubtedly be a boon to families that include these stricken children. This book should be of great importance to the layperson and the professional alike.

After dealing with this problem for the last forty years, I have watched with great anticipation the fear of coma, shock, and, at times, self-destruction.

In most cases this involves the child who rebels against monotonous routines. He longs for pleasing meals that are both palatable and fulfilling. The most important areas seem to be for attractive breakfasts, vegetables, treats, and away-from-home substitutions. I suggest strongly that the identification tag should be worn especially in this day of drug-oriented society.

I truly believe that Mrs. Babington as a concerned parent with dedication does just this. My hat is off to her!

Charles A. Carabello, M.D., F.A.A.P., F.R.S.H.
Formerly Chief of Pediatrics
in The St. Joseph's Hospital
and Community General Hospital
Reading, Pa.

CONTENTS

DISHES INDICATED WITH AN ASTERISK (*)
MAY BE LOCATED IN THE INDEX

PREFACE

Welcome to the healthy world of the diabetic. It is a healthy world because the nature of the disease requires the diabetic to eat a diet that is nutritionally sound. It is also a healthy world for members of the diabetic's family who are served the same foods that the diabetic must eat.

My introduction to the diabetic diet came as abruptly as did the diabetes that caused my daughter to be hospitalized. Her hospital stay lasted for two weeks, during which time we both learned how to stick a "needle" into an orange (a practice run for the daily insulin injections that were to become a part of her life), and I was briefly instructed on the six food exchanges upon which a diabetic diet is based. When Sherry was released from the hospital, I was provided with a list of the amounts of each of the exchanges that she was to eat daily.

And, thus, I came to cook my first diabetic dinner. I waded through the maze of exchanges, and several hours later, still utterly confused, I served each member of my family 2 meat exchanges, 1 fat exchange, 2 fruit exchanges, 1 vegetable exchange, 1 bread exchange, and ½ milk exchange. Needless to say, they were not overjoyed at the prospect of a meal composed of 2 ounces of tuna, ½ cup of carrots, 1 slice of bread, 1 teaspoon of butter, 1 cup of water-packed fruit cocktail, and ½ cup of skim milk.

I had a position as a home economist for a local utility company and I really did not have the time or the inclination to prepare two different dinners. We all ate the same diabetic fare and it was unbelievably monotonous. No wonder diabetics have a difficult time adhering to their diets. But did it have to be so dull?

Taste means more than anything else in food enjoyment, and there are only four tastes: bitter, sour, sweet, and salt. They provide the entire range of food pleasures that we know. Why, then, should meals for the diabetic be any less enjoyable than meals for the most fastidious gourmet? Why couldn't the exchanges be combined in a variety of ways to produce a variety of dishes that my whole family could eat and enjoy? So I started on a totally new experience, full of apprehension, full of confusion, and full of questions for which I hoped to find answers. I was the parent of a diabetic child and the responsibility seemed monumental. There were many obstacles to overcome; there was much to be learned; there was so much that was new and sometimes frightening to me that I wondered if I would ever be able to successfully fulfill my role as the mother of a diabetic. Today, I can look back at the experience with a sense of satisfaction and at an undertaking that proved to be worth all the effort it required, for Sherry is now a happy, healthy, young adult who leads a normal, active life. She is living on a balanced diet that is giving her the nourishment essential to good health and well-being and which allows her body to work at the peak of its potential. It was not always so!

With the onset of her diabetes, Sherry went through a variety of stages. At times she would gorge on ice cream, cake, or cookies. It took a sign on her back saying "Please do not feed me" to keep friends and neighbors from succumbing to her plea for a tasty treat. Then, if she could not have what she wanted, she would not eat anything. Insulin shock was not an uncommon experience. At other times she would overindulge in all kinds of foods until she was so overweight that I wanted to stick her with a pin in hopes of deflating her and bringing her back to her proper size. She kept food hidden in her closet, her chest of drawers, and under her bed. It was not long before she was sharing her room with ants and mice. My sweet, loving child was no longer a joy and a delight. She went through phases of being withdrawn, irritable, angry, and somewhat confused. Then, like Jekyll and Hyde, she would adhere to her diet and become her old dear self.

I was not aware of the inner turmoil that she was suffering. Sherry had been coping with diabetes for ten years, before she was able to share her feelings, about becoming diabetic, with me. This only came about after she first shared her feelings with a newfound friend, also a juvenile diabetic. When Sherry discovered that both she and Diane had gone through the same mental confusion, she began to understand her own reactions. She no longer felt guilty for having hated me and for having blamed me for her illness. She had also blamed her father, whose hobby was gourmet cooking, her grandmother's cook, who made unbelievably rich cookies and confections, and God. Fortunately, today she only blames the sugar industry. She also understands and accepts her dietary limitations and can even think positively about being diabetic. She is actually healthier than most of her peers, who still consume mounds of "junk food."

This change in attitude did not occur overnight. It only came about after she began to realize that she was not so different and that she could eat most of the foods that her friends enjoyed. It did not take me long, after receiving her prescribed daily exchange allowance from her physician, to realize that eating for a diabetic child could be incredibly dull—but it did not have to be! So much could be done to normalize meals and make them interesting, just by combining the exchanges in a variety of different ways. So with a spirit of adventure and a degree in foods and nutrition, I set out to make every day's eating a delightful experience.

Midmorning hunger pains are experienced by anyone who does not eat an adequate, well-balanced breakfast. The fastest cure is a nonnutritional snack, but this is not an acceptable solution for the diabetic. I made sure that the day started with a hearty breakfast, so that Sherry's midmorning thoughts of food would be limited to a curiosity about the contents of her lunch box. Packing her lunch became a daily challenge. I tried to make it interesting and full of surprises. I had visions of her dumping the whole thing into the nearest trash can and spending her allowance on "forbidden foods." Quite naturally the foods that she enjoyed the most were desserts and snacks. A piece of cake had often served as a reward for good behavior. The traditional ball game or after-movie snacks were as important as the actual events themselves. As I continued to experiment with recipes, I discovered many desserts, snacks, and confections that could be prepared from her allotted exchanges. They were also tasty enough to be enjoyed by the whole family.

At times juvenile diabetes can be harder on the parents than their diabetic child. And so to ease your task, I would like to share my experience with you. I hope my recipes will keep your child's eating more normal and more fun. Serve them to your whole family, and you may all benefit. Remember: Good Nutrition=Good Health.

COOKING CREATIVELY FOR YOUR DIABETIC CHILD

DIET AND INSULIN THERAPY

Diabetes is a national health problem affecting 10 million Americans. Ten to 15 percent of the known diabetics are juvenile diabetics. There are two types of diabetes, juvenile-onset diabetes and maturity-onset diabetes. Their classification is derived from the time of life when the diabetes occurs. It is possible for an adult to develop juvenile-onset diabetes and for a child to develop maturity-onset diabetes, but such cases are unusual. The basic cause of diabetes is unknown, but it is brought about by the malfunctioning of the pancreas, a gland located behind the stomach. One of its functions is to produce insulin, a hormone that regulates the body's use of sugar. Insulin enables the body to utilize sugar and to convert it to energy. Without it the sugar cannot be utilized, and thus it accumulates in the body. Juvenile-onset diabetes is the more severe form. Juvenile diabetics have virtually no ability to produce their own insulin and therefore require insulin therapy on a daily basis. In maturity-onset diabetes the pancreas produces some insulin, but the amount is not sufficient to meet the body's requirements. Maturity-onset diabetes is controlled by diet alone or by diet and oral medication. The development of maturity-onset diabetes is gradual and is evidenced by increased hunger, weight loss, and a general feeling of lassitude. The onset of juvenile diabetes is somewhat abrupt. The child may lose consciousness; develop a weak and rapid pulse; be feverish and flushed; and develop dry skin. Teenagers will evidence great thirst, excessive hunger, marked increase in urination, weight loss, general weakness, and fatigue. If untreated, the juvenile diabetic will lapse into a diabetic coma—a condition that requires immediate medical attention.

In the case of the juvenile diabetic there is only one acceptable drug, insulin. It is the only drug that works. Prior to its discovery in 1921, juvenile diabetics had a very short life expectancy and spent most of the time in a semiresponsive state. Insulin has markedly increased their life-span, enabling them to lead a fuller and more normal life, relatively free of complications. Insulin along with proper nutrition is the foundation upon which a juvenile diabetic depends for survival. Together they do the job; alone they are useless.

It is of the utmost importance in the control of your child's diabetes to constantly maintain his blood sugar as close to normal as possible. Essentially, what you are doing is keeping your child's body chemistry regulated so that his body functions similar to the way it would function if he did not have diabetes. Insulin and diet are partners in the treatment of juvenile diabetes; diet therapy sustains the insulin treatment. Without proper diet, the whole support system collapses. There must be a proper balance between the amount of prescribed insulin and the number of calories consumed. The diabetic diet is simply a healthy pattern for eating ordinary foods in controlled amounts at regularly spaced intervals. For best nutrition, feed your child a variety of foods. As we get our minerals and vitamins from a variety of sources, limiting our eating to a few foods limits our mineral and vitamin intake. Large quantities are not necessary; small amounts of foods will provide the desired results. Fresh fruits and vegetables in season are most beneficial.† A variety of meat, fish, and poultry is advisable. Children tend to prefer ground beef and chicken, but you can play a game of introducing new foods into their diet, making it an adventure in good eating. Good nutrition is a way to keep your whole family in the optimum of health. Good nutrition is life-preserving for the diabetic child. It will become a habit for any diabetic, who abides by the rules established by the exchanges. It is a very simple matter to become nutritionally aware. The importance of good nutrition will become more pronounced as you continue to familiarize yourself with your child's diabetic needs. All of us could benefit from the diabetic's diet; it is basically just sound nutrition without any sugar. Too much sugar is not advantageous for anyone, but it is prohibited entirely in the diabetic's diet.

† See Appendixes D and E.

Life without sugar can be their salvation. Sugar is a food that is not harmful in moderation to nondiabetics, but it is never a necessity.

As a parent you have a responsibility to make your child knowledgeable in all pertinent information relating to his diabetic condition. Knowledge will be his personal ally in dealing with diabetes. Lack of knowledge will only add to the confusion he may already be experiencing. Your child should understand that he must assist his body consciously and externally to do what most children's bodies do automatically. With proper instruction, most children accept their diabetes, soon learn to inject themselves with insulin, and generally follow guidelines set down for them. Your diabetic child must realize that he is not different from his peers. However, he does have the responsibility of always practicing self-discipline in his eating habits in order to keep his body functioning normally. As a parent you will have to exercise extreme care and tolerance in helping him to understand his diet. Instill pride in him for his accomplishments in adhering to his prescribed exchanges.

Your diabetic child may experience a reaction to either too low or too high a blood sugar level, conditions that both need immediate treatment. The most common is low blood sugar or insulin (shock) reaction. Once injected, the absorption of insulin into the bloodstream and the simultaneous lowering of blood sugar continue without any relation to the needs of the diabetic. A meal delayed or missed can cause the blood sugar level to drop below the normal level. The symptoms of insulin (shock) reaction are tremors, palpitations, headache, excessive perspiration, and mental confusion. A piece of sugar, a glass of orange juice, or a chocolate bar will eliminate the symptoms in minutes. It is better to err on the side of too much sugar and treat the symptoms, rather than taking a chance on their becoming progressively worse. Diabetics can experience insulin (shock) reaction anytime, anywhere, so it is important that your child carry a small amount of some form of sugar with him at all times.

A high blood sugar level is brought about by insufficient insulin, a condition that usually occurs when a diabetic fails to take insulin or seriously neglects his diet. The resulting problem is a diabetic coma and the diabetic requires immediate medical treatment for proper administration of carefully controlled doses of insulin.

Your diabetic child should have some form of identification to let others know that he is an *insulin-taking diabetic*. A medical card is a help and it should state your child's name and address, doctor's name, and treatment for certain emergencies. Many diabetics wear a tag or a bracelet. They are easier to carry than a card and are more likely to be found by another person. A boy's objections to wearing such a tag can be overcome by pointing out to him that soldiers wear "dog tags" around their necks. If he wants to be a "good soldier," he should always wear his tag. Girls usually like to wear necklaces or bracelets, so you should not have a problem with your daughter. Medical alert tags or bracelets can be purchased from your local jeweler. Or your physician will tell you how to contact the Medic Alert Foundation, a nonprofit organization that will maintain your child's medical records for the duration of his life for an initial fee of ten dollars. He will receive an identification card that will be renewed annually. He will also receive a necklace or a bracelet that will have a medical insignia on the front and will identify your child and his medical condition on the back. A toll-free telephone number will also be engraved on the tag. By calling the medical alert number, his medical information will be made known. This service is available on a twenty-four-hour-a-day basis, every day of the year.

Don't try to keep your child's diabetic condition a secret. Relatives and neighbors should be cautioned not to give in to his entreaties for sweets or unauthorized snacks. All school personnel who have contact with your child should be aware of his diabetes and should know how to recognize and handle insulin reactions. His teacher should have some form of sugar or candy readily available. You can help your child by providing information to the school staff on diabetes, information that is available at no charge in attractive and easily read pamphlets from the

American Diabetes Association, Inc.
600 Fifth Avenue
New York, N.Y. 10020

Treat your diabetic child as you treat all other children. Diabetes is no barrier to living a full and happy life. With proper diet and insulin therapy, your child can grow up to follow most any career of his choosing. Research is always continuing and many great breakthroughs may lay ahead for the diabetic. There are new drugs being developed. A system for monitoring the flow of insulin into the body is being researched. It would regulate the insulin so that the body would always have the proper amount to take care of the sugar that has to be absorbed. At present there is no way to keep the blood sugar constant on any other than a twenty-four hour period. Other promising areas of research include transplantation of healthy insulin cells, an artificial pancreas, and pancreas transplants. A breakthrough in any of these areas will be monumental!

BREAKFAST

Breakfast is the most important meal of the day. Our bodies have been without food for a long period of time and they must be refueled in order to meet the energy needs of the day that is beginning. To skip breakfast is a serious mistake for anyone, but it is not permissible for the diabetic. Your child must start his day with sufficient food to balance his body chemistry with his insulin intake. A well-balanced breakfast is also important to provide the nutrients necessary to keep him functioning at his optimum energy level until lunchtime. Protein foods are especially important in the morning. They have a lasting quality not found in other foods. Breakfast may be a meal enjoyed by the family together, or if your child is ill or in a hurry it may be just a nutritional drink. Nor must breakfast consist of the conventional bacon and eggs. A hamburger and a cup of tomato soup is just as acceptable. How it is eaten is not important; what is important is that it is eaten. It is not advisable to allow your child to skip his prescribed breakfast exchanges, unless you are providing a midmorning snack.

BREAKFAST BEVERAGES

Beverages suitable for breakfast can be found in the chapter on beverages. A glass of skim milk is always acceptable, but for variety you might like to try:

Banana Milk Shake*   Orange Milk Shake*
Hot Chocolate*   Tomato Bouillon*
Cocoa*   Tomato Soup*
Nutrition Snack*   Vegetable Cocktail*
Orange Frost*

FRUITS AND FRUIT JUICES

The Exchange List for Fruits (see Appendix B) will provide you with a wide variety of fruits and juices to serve to your child at breakfast.

CEREALS

The Exchange List for Breads (see Appendix B) will provide you with a list of prepared cereals that are acceptable to serve to your diabetic child. It does not offer a large variety, because most prepared cereals contain an excessive amount of sugar and are not suitable for your purposes. There are a number of easy-to-prepare hot cereals available and ½ cup=1 bread exchange. For variety serve them with ½ small sliced banana, or ½ cup berries in season, or 2 tablespoons raisins. Add 1 fruit exchange.

CORNED BEEF HASH

SERVES 4

(1 serving=2 meat exchanges, 1 fat exchange, and 1 bread exchange)

1 cup chopped canned corned   1 small onion, grated
   beef   3 tablespoons beef broth
2 cups diced well-cooked potatoes

Mix corned beef, potatoes, and onion and chill. Heat beef broth in skillet and place hash in a layer in the bottom of the pan.

Cook over a low flame for 15 minutes. Raise flame to brown hash.

BAKED EGGS IN TOAST CUPS

Preheat oven to 350° F.   SERVES 6

(1 serving=1 meat exchange, 1 fat exchange, and 1 bread exchange)

3 teaspoons butter	6 eggs
6 slices bread	Salt and pepper to taste

Grease each of 6 muffin cups with ½ teaspoon butter. Remove crusts from bread. Press bread into greased cups. Drop 1 egg into each cup. Season with salt and pepper. Bake for 12 minutes or until the eggs are set.

BAKED EGGS AND TOMATO

Preheat oven to 375° F.   SERVES 4

(1 serving=1 vegetable exchange, 1 meat exchange, and 1½ fat exchanges)

2 large tomatoes	4 eggs
Salt and pepper to taste	4 teaspoons butter

Slice tomatoes and place in a lightly greased baking dish or individual ramekins. Season with salt and pepper. Bake for 4 minutes. Break eggs on top of tomato slices. Top with butter and bake for 8 minutes.

BOILED EGGS AND HAM

SERVES 4

(1 serving=2 meat exchanges and 1½ fat exchanges)

4 soft-cooked Eggs*
4 1-ounce slices boiled ham
2 teaspoons butter

Remove eggs from shells and serve on ham slices. Top each with
½ teaspoon butter.

CODDLED EGGS

(1 egg=1 meat exchange and ½ fat exchange)

Immerse the eggs in boiling water, cover the pan, and turn off
the heat. In 8 minutes the whites will be soft and the yolks just
set. In 20 minutes the yolks will be firm and the whites still soft.

POACHED EGGS

(1 egg=1 meat exchange and ½ fat exchange)

Bring 1 cup salted water to a boil. Break the egg into a small
saucer and slide it into the water. Reduce heat and cook for 3
minutes or until the white is firm. The water should not boil.
Remove the egg with a slotted spoon.

For variety, eggs may be poached in milk, consommé, bouillon, or tomato juice.

EGG SAUCERS

Preheat oven to 375° F.   SERVES 4

(1 serving=1 bread exchange, 1 meat exchange, and 1½ fat exchanges)

4 slices bread	**4 eggs**
4 teaspoons butter	**Salt and pepper to taste**

Remove the crust from the bread and butter each slice with 1 teaspoon butter. Place bread on baking sheet and bake for 5 minutes. Break an egg onto each slice of bread. Season with salt and pepper and bake for 8 minutes.

SHIRRED EGGS

(1 egg=1 meat exchange and 1½ fat exchanges)

Melt 1 teaspoon butter in an individual ramekin. Add 1 egg and grill 4 inches from the broiler flame.

Shirred eggs may also be baked with 1 ounce of boiled ham and a round of toast in the bottom of the ramekin. Add 1 meat exchange, ½ bread exchange, and ½ fat exchange.

SCRAMBLED EGGS

SERVES 4

(1 serving=1 meat exchange and 1½ fat exchanges)

4 eggs	Salt and pepper to taste
4 tablespoons skim milk	4 teaspoons butter

Beat eggs with milk and seasoning until well blended. Melt butter in skillet over a low flame. Pour egg mixture into pan and cook stirring constantly, until eggs are firm.

For variety, add 2 ounces chipped beef or 2 ounces chopped ham to eggs before cooking. Add ½ meat exchange per serving for chipped beef. Add ½ meat exchange and ¼ fat exchange for chopped ham.

SOFT-COOKED EGGS

(1 egg=1 meat exchange and ½ fat exchange)

Never boil eggs. Cook them slowly in water below the boiling point. Soft-cooked eggs with firm whites and running yolks take 2 or 3 minutes, depending on the size of the egg. Cook them 2 or 3 minutes longer for very firm whites and yolks that hold their shape. Eggs should be at room temperature before being immersed in hot water. They may be started in cold water and slowly brought to a simmer. This is the same as cooking them for 2 or 3 minutes in hot water.

FLUFFY OMELET

SERVES 4

(1 serving=1 meat exchange and ½ fat exchange)

4 eggs, separated   ½ teaspoon salt
4 tablespoons water   Dash pepper

Beat egg whites until stiff. Mix egg yolks, water, and seasonings and beat slightly. Fold the mixture slowly into the beaten whites. Turn into lightly greased skillet and cook slowly until puffy and browned on bottom. Turn and cook just enough to lightly brown the other side.

POTATO OMELET

SERVES 4

(1 serving=1¾ fat exchanges, ¼ bread exchange, and 1½ meat exchanges)

4 teaspoons butter   Salt and pepper to taste
1 cup cubed cooked potatoes   6 tablespoons grated Parmesan
4 eggs   cheese
1 tablespoon water

Melt butter in skillet, add the potatoes, and cook until they begin to brown. Beat eggs well with water and season with salt and pepper. Pour over potatoes and cook until beginning to set. Sprinkle in the cheese and continue cooking until brown on the bottom.

BLUEBERRY MUFFINS

Preheat oven to 350° F.   YIELDS 8 MUFFINS

(1 muffin=¾ fat exchange, ¼ fruit exchange, and ¾ bread
exchange)

1 egg
¾ cup plain yogurt (made from
   skim milk)
2 tablespoons vegetable oil
1 teaspoon granulated sugar
   substitute (substitute for 4
   tablespoons sugar)

¼ teaspoon salt
1 teaspoon baking soda
¾ cup blueberries
1 cup flour

Mix egg, yogurt, oil, sweetener, and salt until well blended. Stir
in baking soda. Add blueberries. Add flour and mix until well
blended. Bake in greased muffin pan for 30 minutes.

BOLOGNA CHEESE MUFFINS

SERVES 4

(1 serving=2 meat exchanges, 2 fat exchanges, and 1 bread
exchange)

2 English muffins, split
4 1-ounce slices bologna
4 1-ounce slices cheese

Toast muffins. Top each half with a slice of bologna and a slice
of cheese. Broil until cheese melts and browns slightly.

CORN MUFFINS

Preheat oven to 350° F. YIELDS 8 MUFFINS

(1 muffin=1½ bread exchanges, ¾ fat exchange, and ¼ milk exchange)

1 egg
1½ cups yogurt (made from skim milk)
2 tablespoons oil
¾ teaspoon granulated sugar substitute (substitute for 3 tablespoons sugar)

½ teaspoon salt
½ teaspoon baking soda
1½ cups cornmeal

Mix egg, yogurt, oil, sweetener, and salt until well blended. Stir in baking soda. Add cornmeal and mix until smooth. Allow mixture to stand for 5 minutes. Bake in greased muffin tin for 20 minutes.

MUFFIN BURGERS

SERVES 4

(1 serving=1 bread exchange, 2¼ meat exchanges, 1 fat exchange, and ¼ vegetable exchange)

2 English muffins, split
8 ounces lean ground beef
1 egg

½ teaspoon salt
Dash pepper
4 tomato slices

Toast muffins. Mix beef, egg, and seasonings and spread each half muffin with beef mixture. Top with tomato. Broil for 7 minutes.

PANCAKES

SERVES 4

(1 serving=¼ milk exchange, ¼ meat exchange, 1½ fat
exchanges, and 1½ bread exchanges)

1 cup flour	½ teaspoon salt
¼ teaspoon granulated sugar	1 egg, beaten
substitute (substitute for 1	1 cup skim milk
tablespoon sugar)	2 tablespoons butter, melted
1 teaspoon baking powder	

Sift flour, sweetener, baking powder, and salt together. Gradually add egg, milk, and butter. Beat until smooth. Pour batter onto hot, lightly greased griddle or skillet. Cook until bubbles appear on the surface. Turn and brown on the other side.

For buttermilk pancakes substitute 1 cup buttermilk made from skim milk for 1 cup plain skim milk and add 1 teaspoon baking sóda.

Serve pancakes with:

Strawberry Sauce*
Orange Sauce*
or
Fresh Berries in Season*

APPLE PANCAKES

SERVES 3

(1 serving=⅓ fruit exchange, ½ fat exchange, ⅓ meat exchange, 1 bread exchange, and ¼ milk exchange)

½ cup flour
Pinch salt
1 egg
⅔ cup skim milk
1 teaspoon butter, melted
1 apple, sliced

⅛ teaspoon granulated sugar substitute (substitute for 1 teaspoon sugar)
1 tablespoon water
Lemon wedges

Sift flour and salt together. Gradually add egg, ⅓ cup milk, and butter. Beat until smooth. Stir in remaining milk. Pour batter onto a hot, lightly greased griddle or skillet and cook pancakes until bubbles appear on the surface. Turn and brown on the other side. For the filling combine apple, sweetener, and water. Cook slowly to a soft puree. Use to fill pancakes. Roll and serve with lemon wedges.

BLUEBERRY PANCAKES

SERVES 6

(1 serving=⅓ fruit exchange, 1 bread exchange, ½ fat exchange, and ¼ milk exchange)

1 cup flour
¾ teaspoon granulated sugar substitute (substitute for 3 tablespoons sugar)

1 egg, separated
1¼ cups skim milk
1 cup blueberries
1 tablespoon butter, melted

Mix together flour, sweetener, egg yolk, milk, and blueberries. Stir until well blended. Add butter and fold in stiffly beaten egg white. Pour batter onto hot, lightly greased griddle or skillet. Cook pancakes until bubbles appear on the surface. Turn and brown on the other side.

POPOVERS

Preheat oven to 400° F.   YIELDS 12 POPOVERS

(1 popover=½ bread exchange, ¼ meat exchange, and ⅓ fat exchange)

1 cup flour
½ teaspoon salt
3 eggs, beaten

1 cup skim milk
2½ teaspoons butter, melted

Sift flour and salt together. Combine eggs, milk, and melted butter. Gradually add liquid ingredients to dry ingredients and beat until smooth. Pour into well-greased muffin tins. Bake for 40 minutes. Serve hot.

CINNAMON TOAST

SERVES 4

(1 serving=1 bread exchange and 1 fat exchange)

4 teaspoons butter, melted
1 teaspoon cinnamon
½ teaspoon granulated sugar substitute (substitute for 2 tablespoons sugar)

4 slices bread, toasted

Combine butter, cinnamon, and sweetener and spread on toast.

FRENCH TOAST

SERVES 4

(1 serving=2 bread exchanges, ½ meat exchange, and 1¼ fat exchanges)

2 eggs
½ teaspoon salt
1 teaspoon granulated sugar substitute (substitute for 4 tablespoons sugar)

¾ cup skim milk
8 slices bread
4 teaspoons butter

Beat eggs with salt, sweetener, and milk. Dip each slice of bread in egg mixture. Melt butter in skillet and cook bread slices until lightly browned on both sides.

SCHOOL LUNCHES

Diabetes can be a problem when it comes to packing school lunches, but then so are other meals. It will always be a challenge to keep your child's eating a source of enjoyment. Just remember that no matter what meal you are preparing, the rules are always the same. You must follow the prescribed exchanges; there is no other way. The exchanges are the same no matter where they are eaten.

Try a variety as you plan daily meals, especially with those lunches that are eaten at school. There is no supervision, so they must be a treat that you know your child will be anxious to eat. If it does not tempt the palate, it may not be consumed. Use foods that your child enjoys and plan for some surprises that will be a lot of fun.

Young children will find carrying their lunch a novelty and may even want to be involved in the menu planning. Shopping for a lunch box can be a good way to embark on this project. An occasional new lunch box will add variety. That which is regimented can become dull.

Now, I can give you recipes, but you must do the rest. Mix and match to achieve variety. Try to make each day a little different. Soup, sandwich, beverage, and a snack is a good basic rule. Add a piece of fruit or a raw vegetable or two. How you use the allotted exchanges is entirely up to you. Just try to keep things novel in everything you do.

SAMPLE SCHOOL LUNCHES

Meatball Stew*
Cucumber and Radish Sandwich*
Hand Fruit
Date Cookies*
Skim Milk

Chicken and Orange Salad*
Lettuce Leaves (in a plastic bag)
Graham Crackers with Cream Cheese*
Chocolate Pudding*
Skim Milk

Cold Meat Sandwich*
Carrot and Raisin Salad*
Chocolate Cupcakes*
Pink Lemonade*

Hot Tangy Bouillon*
Egg Salad Sandwich*
Potato Chips
Apple Rolls*

SANDWICHES

Sandwiches for school lunches can be prepared in advance and
stored in the freezer. However, you cannot freeze lettuce, tomatoes,
or hard-cooked eggs. Use different types of bread to add variety.
Pocket breads and hard and soft rolls are enjoyed by most children.

SANDWICH FILLINGS

BAKED BEAN

(1 sandwich=3 bread exchanges)

Mash ¼ cup baked beans with Catsup* or Chili Sauce*. Spread on pumpernickel bread and top with another slice of bread.

BANANA AND COTTAGE CHEESE

(1 sandwich=1 fruit exchange, ½ meat exchange, and 2 bread exchanges)

Mash ½ small banana with 1 teaspoon lemon juice. Spread on raisin bread. Top with 2 tablespoons low-fat cottage cheese and another slice of bread.

CARROT AND CELERY

(1 sandwich=1 vegetable exchange, 1 fat exchange, and 2 bread exchanges)

Combine ¼ cup chopped cooked carrots with ¼ cup chopped celery and 1 teaspoon mayonnaise. Spread on whole wheat bread and top with another slice of bread.

CARROT AND PEA

(1 sandwich=½ vegetable exchange, 1 fat exchange, and 2½ bread exchanges)

Combine ½ cup cooked carrots and peas with 1 teaspoon mayonnaise. Spread on white bread and top with another slice of bread.

CHEESE

(1 sandwich=2 meat exchanges, 2 fat exchanges, and 2 bread exchanges)

Place 2 ounces Swiss or Cheddar type cheese between 2 slices of rye bread that have been spread with mustard.

CHEESE AND NUT

(1 sandwich=1 meat exchange, 1 fat exchange, and 2 bread exchanges)

Combine 4 tablespoons low-fat cottage cheese with 6 chopped walnuts. Spread on whole wheat bread and top with another slice of bread.

CHICKEN SALAD

(1 sandwich=1 meat exchange, ½ vegetable exchange, 1 fat exchange, and 2 bread exchanges)

Combine 1 ounce chopped cooked chicken with ¼ cup chopped celery and 1 teaspoon mayonnaise. Spread on white bread and top with lettuce leaves and another slice of bread.

CHICKEN AND TOMATO

(1 sandwich=1 meat exchange, 1 fat exchange, 2 bread exchanges, and ¼ vegetable exchange)

Spread 2 slices bread with 1 teaspoon mayonnaise. Arrange 1 ounce sliced chicken, 1 tomato slice, and 2 lettuce leaves on 1 slice of bread. Top with remaining slice of bread.

CORNED BEEF

(1 sandwich=1 meat exchange, 1½ fat exchanges, and 2 bread exchanges)

Spread 2 slices rye or pumpernickel bread with 1 teaspoon mayonnaise. Arrange 1 ounce canned corned beef and 4 dill pickle slices on 1 slice of bread. Top with 2 lettuce leaves and remaining slice of bread.

CUCUMBER AND RADISH

(1 sandwich=½ vegetable exchange, 1 fat exchange, and 2 bread exchanges)

Spread 2 slices whole wheat bread with 1 teaspoon mayonnaise. Arrange ¼ cup thinly sliced cucumbers on 1 slice of bread. Top with radish slices. Season with salt and pepper and top with remaining slice of bread.

EGG SALAD

(1 sandwich=1 meat exchange, 1½ fat exchanges, and 2 bread exchanges)

Combine 1 chopped hard-cooked egg with 1 teaspoon mayonnaise, ¼ teaspoon vinegar, and a dash of salt and pepper. Mash into a smooth paste. Spread on 1 slice whole wheat bread. Top with 4 slices raw carrot, 4 slices dill pickle, and another slice of bread.

EGG AND TOMATO

(1 sandwich=½ vegetable exchange, ½ meat exchange, 1¼ fat exchanges, and 2 bread exchanges)

Spread 2 slices bread with 1 teaspoon mayonnaise. Arrange 2 lettuce leaves, 2 tomato slices, and ½ sliced hard-cooked egg on 1 slice of bread. Season with salt and pepper and top with remaining slice of bread.

HAM AND CHICKEN SALAD

(1 sandwich=1 meat exchange, 1¼ fat exchanges, 2 bread exchanges, and ½ vegetable exchange)

Combine ½ ounce boiled ham, ½ ounce chopped chicken, ¼ cup chopped celery, and 1 teaspoon mayonnaise. Spread mixture on 1 slice of bread. Top with lettuce leaves and another slice of bread.

HAM AND EGG

(1 sandwich=1½ meat exchanges, 2¼ fat exchanges, and 2 bread exchanges)

Combine 1 ounce deviled ham, ½ chopped hard-cooked egg, and 1 teaspoon mayonnaise. Season to taste with salt and pepper and spread on hard sandwich roll.

HAM AND PEANUT BUTTER

(1 sandwich=1½ meat exchanges, 2¼ fat exchanges, and 2 bread exchanges)

Combine 1 ounce deviled ham, 1 tablespoon peanut butter, and ½ teaspoon mustard. Spread on raisin bread and top with another slice of bread.

LEBANON BOLOGNA

(1 sandwich=1 meat exchange, 1 fat exchange, and 1 bread exchange)

Fill small pocket bread with 1 ounce Lebanon bologna and top with Catsup*.

LIVERWURST

(1 sandwich=1 meat exchange, 2 fat exchanges, and 2 bread exchanges)

Combine 1 ounce liverwurst with 1 teaspoon mayonnaise and 1 teaspoon minced onion. Spread on rye bread and top with another slice of bread.

COLD MEAT

(1 sandwich=1 meat exchange, 1½ fat exchanges, and 2 bread exchanges)

Arrange 1 ounce leftover cold meat on a soft roll. Spread with 1 teaspoon mayonnaise. Top with pickle slices and lettuce leaves.

MEAT LOAF

(1 sandwich=1 meat exchange, ½ fat exchange, and 2 bread exchanges)

Spread 2 slices rye bread with mustard. Arrange 1 ounce meat loaf on 1 slice of bread and top with remaining slice.

TONGUE AND COLESLAW

(1 sandwich=1 meat exchange, 1½ fat exchanges, ½ vegetable exchange, and 2 bread exchanges)

Spread 2 slices rye bread with 1 teaspoon mayonnaise. Arrange 1 ounce sliced tongue on bread. Top with ¼ cup Coleslaw* and remaining slice of bread.

TUNA SALAD

(1 sandwich=1 meat exchange, 1 fat exchange, and 2 bread exchanges)

Mix ¼ cup tuna with 1 teaspoon mayonnaise, 1 teaspoon lemon juice, 1 tablespoon chopped celery, and 1 tablespoon green pepper. Spread on soft sandwich roll.

HOT LUNCHES

On cold wintry days your child will enjoy a hot food in his lunch box. A wide-mouth thermos will enable you to package hot soups or entrées. Make extra portions for dinner and freeze them for future lunches. Soups may also be prepared in advance and stored in the freezer. Some suggestions for hot lunches that your child will enjoy are:

Beef Bouillon
Beef Noodle Casserole*
Chicken Bouillon*
Hot Tangy Bouillon*
Tomato Bouillon*
Chili*
Fish Chowder*
Macaroni and Cheese*
Spaghetti*
Spanish Rice*

Chili Soup*
Hot Dog Soup*
Peanut Butter Soup*
Tomato Soup*
Vegetable Soup*
Beef Stew*
Hamburger Stew*
Lamb Stew*
Veal Stew*

SNACKS

I have prepared a list of foods from which you may want to choose a little something extra to include with each day's lunch. Something a bit different to add variety, they will make for more interesting meals.

Cheese Cubes: 1 ounce=1 meat exchange and 1 fat exchange.
Oven-fried Chicken*
Corn Chips: 15=1 bread exchange and 2 fat exchanges.
Butter-type Crackers: 5=1 bread exchange and 1 fat exchange.
Deviled Eggs*
Hard-cooked Eggs*: 1 egg=1 meat exchange and ½ fat exchange.
Graham Cracker Snacks*
Marbles*
Blueberry Muffins*
Corn Muffins*
Spanish Peanuts: 20 whole=1 fat exchange.
Peanut Butter Balls*
Pickles (unsweetened): need not be counted as an exchange.
Popcorn*
Potato Chips: 15=1 bread exchange and 2 fat exchanges.
Pretzel Sticks (3⅛"×⅛"): 25=1 bread exchange.
Raisins: 2 tablespoons=1 fruit exchange.
Saltines: 6=1 bread exchange.
Yogurt (made from skim milk): 1 cup=1 milk exchange.

SALADS

Salads are a nice addition to a school lunch box. They add interesting textures and flavors. Try to include some form of salad with each day's lunch. They can be very simple and still provide essential nutrients. Some salad ideas:

Carrot Raisin Salad*
Celery and Carrot Sticks: ½ cup=1 vegetable exchange.
Stuffed Celery*
Coleslaw*
Low-fat Cottage Cheese with Chopped Fruit or Chopped Raw Vegetables: ¼ cup cottage cheese=1 meat exchange; ½ cup fruit=1 fruit exchange; ½ cup vegetables=1 vegetable exchange.
Pickled Cucumber Salad*
Cucumber Sticks: ½ cup=1 vegetable exchange.
Mixed Fruit Salad*
Orange Chicken Salad*
Radishes: need not be counted as an exchange.
Cherry Tomatoes: ½ cup=1 vegetable exchange.
Whole Small Tomato: 1 vegetable exchange.
Waldorf Salad*
Plain Yogurt (made from skim milk) with fruit: 1 cup yogurt=1 milk exchange; ½ cup fruit=1 fruit exchange.

BEVERAGES

Milk is often provided by the school cafeteria. If you are certain that skim milk is available, it will not be necessary to include it in the lunch box. At times your child will enjoy having beverages other than plain milk. For variety you may want to include any of the following:

Spicy Apple Cider*
Apple Juice (unsweetened): ⅓ cup=1 fruit exchange.
Beef broth with Apple Juice (unsweetened): 1 cup beef broth combined with ⅓ cup apple juice and a dash of cinnamon= 1 fruit exchange.
Cocoa*

Artificially Sweetened Cranberry Juice: need not be counted as an exchange.

Grapefruit Juice (unsweetened): ½ cup=1 fruit exchange.

Pink Lemonade*

Orangeade*

Orange Milk Shake*

Pineapple Fizz: ⅓ cup unsweetened pineapple juice, ⅓ cup artificially sweetened cranberry juice, and ⅓ cup artificially sweetened carbonated lemon-lime soda=1 fruit exchange.

Tomato Juice (with dash lemon or lime juice): ½ cup=1 vegetable exchange.

Vegetable Cocktail*

DESSERTS

Desserts are always a *must!* Without dessert a lunch box most certainly will seem incomplete. It is the first thing your child will look for when he opens his lunch box and may well be the first thing he eats.

Some dessert ideas:

1 Small Apple=1 fruit exchange.

Apple Grapefruit Compote*

Apple Rolls*

Applesauce*

1 Small Banana=2 fruit exchanges.

Banana Pudding*

Chocolate Cake*

Chocolate Cupcakes*

Date Cookies*

Baked Custard*

Rice Custard*

Water-packed Canned Fruit: ½ cup=1 fruit exchange.

Fruit-flavored Gelatin: Artificially sweetened gelatin dessert need not be counted as an exchange.

1 Small Orange=1 fruit exchange.

Orange Slices: ½ cup=1 fruit exchange.

1 Medium Peach=1 fruit exchange.

Peaches Melba*

1 Small Pear=1 fruit exchange.

Pear Sauce*
Spiced Pears*
Chocolate Pudding*
Lemon Pudding*
Pineapple Pudding*
Rice Pudding*
Vanilla Pudding*
1 Medium Tangerine=1 fruit exchange.
Watermelon Balls: 1 cup=1 fruit exchange.

SOUPS

Soups are an ideal food for cold winter days, to pack in a thermos for school lunches, to start a meal on a cool summer's day, to be eaten as an entree. They may be served piping hot, ice cold, or jellied. Soups will always play an important role in the diet of diabetic children. They add variety to meals, and children enjoy them, because they are easy to swallow. The old wives' tale of the value of chicken noodle soup is not to be taken lightly; soups are very beneficial when your child is ill.

Make a practice of serving soup as a main dish. Not only is it nutritional, it is also economical and will always stand you and your family in good stead. Diabetic children would do well to develop the soup habit, because they can include as many of the exchanges as you care to use.

Bouillon is a "free food" and therefore I have used it as a base for most soups. With a little imagination you can create your own soups. All you need is a quart of bouillon, the leftovers in the refrigerator that you knew you would find a use for, and a few herbs and spices to enhance the flavor of the finished product.

Jellied soups, stored in a jar in the refrigerator, are ideal for a between-meals pickup.

JELLIED BOUILLON

SERVES 4 TO 6

(need not be counted as an exchange)

1½ tablespoons unflavored gelatin	1 onion, sliced
½ cup cold water	1 small bunch parsley
2 cups beef bouillon	½ teaspoon salt
1 cup chicken bouillon	Dash pepper

Soak gelatin in cold water for 5 minutes. Combine remaining ingredients. Heat to boiling point. Reduce heat and simmer 10 minutes. Add gelatin and stir until dissolved. Let stand 5 minutes. Strain and pour into bouillon cups and chill until firm. Just before serving, draw a fork through the jelly to break it up. Sprinkle with finely chopped chives and garnish with lemon wedges.

Jellied bouillon served in half a cantaloupe on a warm summer's day=2 fruit exchanges.

HOT TANGY BOUILLON*
●
TOMATO BOUILLON

SERVES 4 TO 6

(1 cup=1 vegetable exchange)

2 cups tomato juice	½ teaspoon basil
2 cups beef bouillon	Lemon slices

Combine tomato juice, bouillon, and basil. Heat and serve garnished with lemon slices.

BORSCH

SERVES 4 TO 6

(1 cup=1 vegetable exchange)

2 cups cooked julienne beets	¾ teaspoon granulated sugar
½ cup finely chopped onion	substitute (substitute for 3
2 cups beef bouillon	tablespoons sugar)
2 cups water	¼ cup lemon juice
1 teaspoon salt	Fresh dill

Combine all ingredients except dill. Bring to a boil. Cover, reduce heat, and simmer for 5 minutes. Borsch may be served hot or cold. Garnish with fresh dill.

CLAM BROTH

SERVES 4 TO 6

(1 serving=1 fat exchange if served with butter)

2 quarts unshelled clams
1¾ cups cold water

Wash and scrub clams very thoroughly with a stiff brush. Place clams in water and cook, covered, until they are steamed open. Open clams all the way to secure all of the juice. Strain the liquor through cheesecloth or a very fine sieve. Reheat and add salt if needed. Serve garnished with teaspoon of butter.

If you are going to eat the steamed clams—and they are hard to resist—5 clams=1 meat exchange.

Of course, you will want to dip them in melted butter: 1 teaspoon butter=1 fat exchange.

JELLIED CLAM TOMATO SOUP

SERVES 4

(1 serving=¾ vegetable exchange)

1 envelope unflavored gelatin
1½ cups tomato juice
¾ cup clam broth
¼ teaspoon celery salt

½ teaspoon Worcestershire sauce
⅛ teaspoon Tabasco sauce
2 tablespoons lemon juice

Sprinkle gelatin on ½ cup of the tomato juice to soften. Place over low heat and stir until gelatin is dissolved. Remove from heat and stir in remaining ingredients. Pour into 8-inch-square pan and chill until firm. To serve, cut into cubes and turn into serving dishes. Garnish with lemon slices.

CHILI SOUP

SERVES 4

(1 serving=2 meat exchanges, 1 fat exchange, ¼ milk exchange, and ½ vegetable exchange)

½ pound lean ground beef
2 tablespoons chopped onion
1 teaspoon chili powder

½ teaspoon salt
2 cups Tomato Soup*
2 cups beef bouillon

Combine beef, onion, chili powder, and salt. Shape into 12 meatballs. Sprinkle skillet lightly with salt and sauté meatballs over low flame until brown. Add tomato soup and bouillon and heat.

FISH CHOWDER*
●
GAZPACHO*
●
CREAM OF GREEN PEA SOUP

SERVES 4

(1 serving=¼ vegetable exchange, ¾ milk exchange
and 1 bread exchange)

1½ cups frozen green peas,
 thawed
2 chicken bouillon cubes
½ cup chopped onion

2 tablespoons flour
3 cups skim milk
Dash pepper
Dash mace

Put all ingredients into blender and blend until smooth. Pour into saucepan and cook, stirring constantly, until thickened.

HOT DOG SOUP

SERVES 4

(1 serving=1 meat exchange, 1½ fat exchanges, ¼ milk exchange, ½ vegetable exchange, and ½ bread exchange)

4 hot dogs, thinly sliced
4 tablespoons chopped onion
2 teaspoons butter

2 cups Tomato Soup*
1 cup cooked rice

Brown hot dogs and onion in butter. Add soup and rice and heat.

JULIENNE SOUP

(need not be counted as an exchange)

Bouillon served with cooked carrots, onions, turnip, and celery which have been cut into shreds about as thick as a match. The vegetables should be boiled in clear water before being added to the bouillon. Allow ¾ cup of vegetables to 4 cups bouillon.

MEATBALL SOUP

SERVES 4

(1 serving=2 meat exchanges, 1 fat exchange, 1 vegetable exchange, ¼ milk exchange, and 1½ bread exchanges)

½ pound lean ground beef	½ cup sliced onion
½ cup bread crumbs	½ cup sliced carrots
1 cup skim milk	2 cups water
2½ teaspoons salt	1 cup tomato juice
Dash pepper	1 tablespoon vinegar
2 cups cubed potatoes	

Combine beef, bread crumbs, ½ cup skim milk, ½ teaspoon salt, and pepper. Form into 16 meatballs. In a 3-quart saucepan combine potatoes, onion, carrots, water, and remaining salt. Bring to boil and add meatballs. Cook 30 minutes. Add remaining milk, tomato juice, and vinegar. Skim off any fat before serving.

FRENCH ONION SOUP*
•
PEANUT BUTTER SOUP

SERVES 4

(1 serving=½ milk exchange, ½ meat exchange, and 1¾ fat exchanges)

1 teaspoon minced onion   1 cup chicken bouillon
2 teaspoons butter   2 cups skim milk
¼ cup peanut butter   ¼ teaspoon salt

Sauté onion in butter until lightly browned. Remove from heat and add peanut butter. Stir until smooth. Gradually stir in bouillon and milk and heat. Season with salt.

SPINACH SOUP

SERVES 4

(1 serving=1¾ vegetable exchanges, ¾ milk exchange, and 1 fat exchange)

2 cups chopped fresh spinach   1 tablespoon lemon juice
4 teaspoons butter   ¼ teaspoon nutmeg
3 cups Tomato Soup*

Sauté spinach in butter for 5 minutes. Add remaining ingredients and heat.

TOMATO SOUP

SERVES 4

(1 serving=1 vegetable exchange, ½ milk exchange,
and ¼ bread exchange)

2 cups tomato juice
2 tablespoons chopped onion
3 tablespoons flour
2 cups skim milk
¼ teaspoon granulated sugar
   substitute (substitute for 2
   teaspoons sugar)

1 teaspoon salt
¼ teaspoon garlic salt
Dash pepper
Dash oregano
Dash basil
Dash thyme

Combine tomato juice, onion, and flour in blender. Blend for 20 seconds. Pour into saucepan and bring to a boil, stirring constantly. Boil 1 minute. Add milk and seasonings. Heat.

GREEN VEGETABLE SOUP

SERVES 6

(1 serving=2 vegetable exchanges)

1 cup sliced carrots
1 cup sliced onion
½ cup sliced celery
2 cups shredded cabbage

2 cups French-cut green beans
4 cups chicken bouillon
1 teaspoon salt
½ teaspoon caraway seed

Combine all ingredients and cook for 30 minutes.

WATERCRESS SOUP

SERVES 4

(need not be counted as an exchange)

4 cups beef bouillon
¼ cup minced watercress
2 tablespoons lemon juice

Combine all ingredients and refrigerate at least 4 hours. Serve chilled.

MEAT AND POULTRY

Meats for your diabetic child are best served either roasted or broiled. Some panfrying is also acceptable. Oven frying is a good way to feed your child fried foods without the addition of any fat. Be sure to purchase lean meats or trim any excess fat from the meat before it is cooked.

In purchasing meats it is always advisable to deal with a butcher who will cut your meat to order. In this way you can be certain of the cut of meat you are going to be cooking. Less tender cuts of meat are best roasted; tender cuts can be broiled. Some meats may be boiled and used for stews.

In general, meat cooking falls into four classifications: beef, pork, lamb, and veal. Beef is the most popular of the meats. A good piece of beef is bright red in color, well marbled, and encased in thick white fat. Top quality lamb is pink and fine-textured. The fat is creamy white and crisp. Pork is gaining in popularity and is available all year round. A good piece of pork is a grayish-pink color, is well marbled with white fat, and is firm and fine-grained. Veal comes from a young calf. It should be pink and firm. It should always be well cooked. The most desirable is "milk-fed" veal—veal from calves that have been fed only milk.

A good rule to follow in purchasing meat is to allow ¼ pound (4 ounces) per average serving. You will have to weigh the amount served to your diabetic child so that you can calculate the number of exchanges that are being consumed.

ROAST BEEF

Preheat oven to 325° F.

(1 ounce=1 meat exchange)

All roasts should stand at room temperature for at least 1 hour before roasting. Time schedules for roasting can only be approximated. The size and shape of the roast, as well as the amount of bone, will affect the cooking time. A meat thermometer will ensure you the greatest degree of accuracy. A temperature of 140° will give you a rare roast, 160° a medium roast, and 170° a well-done roast. If you do not have a meat thermometer, allow 18 to 20 minutes per pound for rare roast, 20 to 25 minutes per pound for medium well-done, and 30 minutes per pound for well-done.

PRIME RIBS OF BEEF

Preheat oven to 325° F.   SERVES 6

(1 ounce=1 meat exchange)

Ask your butcher for the first three ribs. Rub the roast with salt and freshly ground pepper. Allow ½ teaspoon of salt per pound. Roast, fat side up, in an uncovered pan. The roast should then rest in the pan at room temperature for about 20 minutes before it is carved.

ROAST FILLET OF BEEF

Preheat oven to 325° F. SERVES 8

(1 ounce=1 meat exchange)

Let stand at room temperature for 1 hour before roasting. Wipe the fillet with a damp cloth. Trim off all of the fat and remove all connective tissue and skin. Season with salt and pepper. Make a bed of chopped celery, lettuce, and onion in the bottom of the roasting pan and place the fillet on top. Roast for 25 to 35 minutes, depending on the size of the roast. The weight of the fillet is usually between 3 and 4 pounds. Baste frequently with hot beef stock for the first 15 minutes and then with pan juices for the remaining time.

BROILED STEAK

(1 ounce=1 meat exchange)

Use tenderloin, sirloin, porterhouse, rib steak, or fillet. Let the steak stand at room temperature for 1 hour. Rub meat with salt and pepper. Place meat on a cold broiler grid and broil 2 to 3 inches from flame. Sear quickly on one side, turn and broil to desired degree of "doneness"—12 minutes for rare, 20 minutes for medium, and 30 minutes for well-done.

BOILED BEEF

SERVES 6 TO 8

(1 ounce beef=1 meat exchange)

1 3-pound boneless beef roast
   (rump, bottom round, or chuck)
3 pounds chicken parts (back,
   wings, giblets, and neck)
2 quarts water
2 teaspoons salt
2 medium onions, quartered
1 parsnip, cut into 1-inch pieces

3 carrots, cut into 1-inch pieces
4 large celery ribs, cut into 1-inch
   pieces
4 sprigs parsley
1 bay leaf
6 peppercorns
¼ teaspoon allspice

In a large soup kettle, combine beef and chicken parts and cover with water. Add salt. Bring to a boil over high heat, adding more water if necessary to cover. Skim off surface scum as it arises. Add vegetables and parsley, bring to a boil, and skim off surface scum. Add bay leaf, peppercorns, and allspice. Lower heat, cover, and simmer for 2 hours. Remove beef to a serving platter. Skim the surface fat from the stock and strain through a sieve. Taste for seasoning. The stock may be served as a soup and need not be counted as an exchange.

BRISKET OF BEEF

SERVES 8

(1 ounce beef=1 meat exchange and 1 fat exchange)
(½ cup cabbage=1 vegetable exchange)
(1 small potato=1 bread exchange)

1 3–3½-pound brisket of beef   1 head cabbage
4 bay leaves   8 small boiled potatoes
1 teaspoon cloves   Horseradish
1 medium onion

Wash brisket of beef under running water and cover the meat with cold water. Bring to a boil and cook for 5 minutes. Skim off surface scum. Cover and simmer for 1 hour. Drain, cover with fresh cold water, and add bay leaves, cloves, and onion. Bring to a boil, lower heat, and simmer until meat is tender. Cool in the stock until it is easy to handle. Slice the long way of the piece of meat and place on a hot platter with just enough stock to keep it moist.

Twelve minutes before you are ready to eat, cut the head of cabbage in eighths, add to the stock, and boil uncovered. Serve with boiled potatoes and horseradish.

Your more sophisticated teenager may enjoy:

BEEF BOURGUIGNON

Preheat oven to 350° F.   SERVES 4

(1 ounce meat=1 meat exchange)
(½ cup vegetables=1 vegetable exchange)

1 pound beef, cut into 1-inch   1 tablespoon tomato paste
   cubes   ¼ teaspoon oregano
1 cup beef bouillon   ¼ teaspoon basil
1 1-pound can small white onions   1 clove garlic, minced
½ pound mushrooms, sliced

Brown meat in a heavy pan in the oven for 20 minutes. Reduce heat to 250° F. Add remaining ingredients, cover, and continue cooking 2 to 3 hours.

BEEF STEW

Preheat oven to 350° F.   SERVES 4 TO 6

(1 ounce meat=1 meat exchange)
(½ cup vegetables=1 vegetable exchange)

2 pounds beef, cut into 1-inch
  cubes
1 teaspoon salt
¼ teaspoon pepper
6 carrots, cut into 1-inch pieces

1 cup sliced celery
1 large onion, sliced
1 clove garlic, minced
1 28-ounce can tomatoes
1 bay leaf

Sprinkle meat with salt and pepper. Brown in a heavy pan in the oven for 20 minutes. When meat is seared, remove from oven and add remaining ingredients. Cover and simmer over a low flame for 1½ hours or until tender.

FLANK STEAK

SERVES 4

(1 ounce meat=1 meat exchange)

1 1-to-1½ pound flank steak
½ cup lemon juice
2 tablespoons soy sauce
¾ teaspoon granulated sugar
  substitute (substitute for 3
  tablespoons sugar)

½ teaspoon salt
⅛ teaspoon oregano

Combine all ingredients and pour over steak. Marinate for 2 hours at room temperature. Remove steak from marinade and broil 3 inches from flame. Allow 5 minutes on each side for rare, 8 minutes for medium, and 10 minutes for well-done. Slice thin on a slant and serve with pan juices.

HAMBURGERS

SERVES 8

(1 serving=2 meat exchanges and 1 fat exchange)

1 pound lean ground beef　　　　¼ teaspoon pepper
1½ teaspoons salt
¾ teaspoon Beau Monde
　seasoning

Mix meat and seasonings and form into 8 patties. Place on cold broiler and broil 3 inches from the flame for 6 minutes on each side.

Hamburger may also be panfried. Sprinkle the bottom of a skillet with salt and cook hamburgers over a low flame.

GRILLED HAMBURGERS*
●
HAMBURGER STEW

SERVES 4

(1 serving=2 meat exchanges, 2 fat exchanges, 1¾ vegetable exchanges, ¾ bread exchange, and ½ milk exchange)

Shaker of salt
½ pound lean ground beef
2 cups tomato juice
½ cup chopped onion
1 cup diced potatoes
1 cup diced carrots

1 tablespoon lemon juice
2 teaspoons salt
4 teaspoons butter
2 tablespoons flour
2 cups milk

Sprinkle bottom of skillet or heavy pan with salt. Add meat and brown over low heat. Drain off excess fat. Add tomato juice, onion, potatoes, carrots, lemon juice, and salt. Cover and simmer for 30 minutes. In a saucepan melt butter and gradually add flour, stirring constantly. Gradually add milk and cook over a low flame for 3 to 5 minutes, stirring constantly. Add white sauce to stew. Serve in soup bowls.

MEATBALLS

Preheat oven to 350° F.   SERVES 4

(1 meatball=1 meat exchange and ½ fat exchange)

1 pound lean ground beef
2 tablespoons bread crumbs
1 egg
½ teaspoon salt
½ cup chopped onion
⅓ cup chopped green pepper
1 cup Tomato Soup*

½ teaspoon granulated brown
  sugar substitute (substitute for 2
  tablespoons brown sugar)
1 tablespoon vinegar
1 tablespoon Worcestershire sauce
1 teaspoon prepared mustard

Mix meat, bread crumbs, egg, and salt. Shape into 16 balls. Place in a shallow baking dish and broil 6 minutes on each side. Pour off fat. Combine remaining ingredients and cook over low heat until blended. Pour over meatballs. Cover and bake for 20 minutes.

MEAT LOAF

Preheat oven to 375° F.   SERVES 4

(1 ounce=1 meat exchange and ½ fat exchange)

1 pound lean ground beef   1 egg
2 tablespoons chopped onion   ½ teaspoon salt
½ cup bread crumbs   1 cup Tomato Sauce*

Combine beef, onion, bread crumbs, egg, and salt. Shape into a loaf. Place in baking dish. Top with tomato sauce and bake for 1 hour.

SHEPHERD'S PIE

Preheat oven to 425° F.   SERVES 4

(1 serving=2 meat exchanges, 1 fat exchange, ¾ vegetable
exchange, and ½ bread exchange)

Shaker of salt   1 cup Tomato Soup*
½ pound lean ground beef   ½ teaspoon salt
¼ cup chopped onion   1 cup mashed potatoes
1 cup cooked mixed vegetables

Sprinkle skillet with salt, add meat and onion, and brown over low flame. Drain off excess fat. Stir in vegetables, soup, and salt. Spoon into casserole, top with mashed potatoes, and bake for 15 minutes.

SHORT RIBS OF BEEF

SERVES 6

(1 ounce meat=1 meat exchange)

6 pounds short ribs
2 medium onions, sliced
1 carrot, cut into 1-inch pieces
1 teaspoon salt

¼ teaspoon pepper
1 tablespoon MSG
Grated horseradish to taste
½ cup chopped parsley

Cover meat with cold water and cook over high heat until water boils. Reduce heat, add onion, carrot, salt, pepper, and MSG, and simmer for 2 hours. Remove ribs to serving platter. Strain broth and season with horseradish. Sprinkle with chopped parsley. Broth need not be counted as an exchange.

SLOPPY JOES*
●
SPAGHETTI

SERVES 4

(1 serving=2 meat exchanges, 3 vegetable exchanges, 2 fat exchanges, and 2 bread exchanges)

½ pound lean ground beef
2 cups sliced mushrooms
4 teaspoons butter
2 cups Tomato Sauce*
4 tomatoes, quartered
1 teaspoon salt

¼ teaspoon basil
¼ teaspoon oregano
4 tablespoons chives
4 tablespoons chopped fresh
  parsley
4 cups cooked spaghetti

CALF'S LIVER

Preheat broiler   SERVES 4

(1 serving=2 meat exchanges, 1 vegetable exchange, and 2 fat exchanges)

8 ounces calf's liver
Salt and pepper to taste
2 tablespoons wine vinegar

2 cups sliced onion
4 teaspoons butter

Season liver with salt and pepper and sprinkle with vinegar. Broil about 5 inches from the flame for 4 minutes on each side. Sauté onion in butter and serve over liver.

IRISH LAMB STEW

SERVES 4

(1 ounce lamb=1 meat exchange; 1 small potato=1 bread exchange; ½ cup peas=1 bread exchange; and ½ cup cabbage=1 vegetable exchange)

1 pound lamb shoulder, cut into
  2-inch cubes
2 onions, quartered
4 carrots
8 small potatoes
1 small head cabbage, cubed

2 tablespoons parsley
2 teaspoons salt
⅛ teaspoon pepper
1 clove garlic, crushed
2 tablespoons lemon juice
2 cups cooked green peas

Cover lamb with water and simmer, skimming off scum as it appears. Add onions and carrots and continue cooking slowly for 1 hour or until meat is tender. Add potatoes and cook 15 minutes longer. Add cabbage and parsley and cook 12 minutes longer. Season with salt, pepper, garlic, and lemon juice and serve sprinkled with peas.

MUTTON CHOPS

Preheat oven to 350° F.   SERVES 4

(1 ounce mutton=1 meat exchange)

4 loin mutton chops   ¼ teaspoon pepper
½ teaspoon salt   Dash garlic salt

Sear chops, on both sides, 2 inches below broiler flame. Season and bake for 20 to 30 minutes.

LEG OF LAMB

Preheat oven to 350° F.   SERVES 8

(1 ounce=1 meat exchange)

1 5–6-pound leg of lamb   ½ cup water
2 cloves garlic   1 medium onion, sliced
Salt and pepper to taste   1 small carrot, sliced

With a sharp knife, puncture a leg of lamb in 5 or 6 different places (top and underside) and insert tiny strips of garlic. Rub meat with salt and pepper. Place in a roasting pan, pour in water, and add onion and carrot. Roast uncovered for 25 minutes per pound. Serve with mint sauce (below).

MINT SAUCE

(need not be counted as an exchange)

1 cup pan drippings from leg of
  lamb (above)
1 tablespoon vinegar

¼ cup low-calorie artificially
  sweetened currant jelly
2 tablespoons chopped fresh mint

Skim fat from pan drippings. Cook drippings, vinegar, and jelly together until jelly is dissolved. Add mint and serve with leg of lamb.

PICKLED FRANKFURTERS*
●
BAKED HAM*
●
ROAST LOIN OF PORK

Preheat oven to 350° F.   SERVES 6

(1 ounce pork=1 meat exchange and ½ fat exchange)

1 4–5-pound loin of pork
Juice of ½ lemon

½ teaspoon salt
2 cups water

Wipe loin of pork with a damp cloth. Rub it with lemon juice and let it stand at room temperature for 15 minutes. Place the loin in a roasting pan, sprinkle it with salt, and add water. Roast for 2½ to 3 hours depending on the size. Cover the pan for the first 30 minutes and then remove the lid.

PORK CHOPS AND APPLESAUCE

SERVES 4

(1 ounce pork=1 meat exchange, and ½ fat exchange; ½ cup
applesauce=1 fruit exchange)

4 loin pork chops	½ teaspoon cinnamon
Salt and pepper to taste	Dash nutmeg
2 cups artificially sweetened	2 teaspoons orange peel
applesauce	

Broil pork chops 3 inches from flame until brown on both sides.
Season with salt and pepper. Remove to skillet. Top with applesauce seasoned with cinnamon, nutmeg, and orange peel. Cover
and simmer 45 minutes.

GERMAN PORK CHOPS

Preheat oven to 350° F.   SERVES 4

(1 ounce pork=1 meat exchange and ½ fat exchange; ½ cup
sauerkraut=1 vegetable exchange; 1 small potato=1 bread
exchange)

Shaker of salt	Salt and pepper to taste
4 loin pork chops	2 cups sauerkraut (with juice)
4 small potatoes, sliced	1 teaspoon caraway seed

Sprinkle skillet with salt, add pork chops, and brown over a low
flame for 5 minutes on each side. Arrange potatoes in the bottom of a baking dish and sprinkle with salt. Top with sauerkraut

and sprinkle with caraway seed. Place pork chops on top of sauerkraut. Sprinkle with salt and pepper. Cover and bake for 1 hour.

ORANGE PINEAPPLE PORK CHOPS

Preheat oven to 350° F. SERVES 4

(1 ounce pork=1 meat exchange and ½ fat exchange; ¼ cup pineapple=½ fruit exchange; ¼ cup orange juice=½ fruit exchange)

Shaker of salt
4 loin pork chops
1 cup crushed unsweetened
  pineapple

1 cup orange juice
Salt to taste

Sprinkle skillet with salt, add pork chops, and brown over a low flame for 5 minutes on each side. Arrange pork chops in a baking dish. Season with salt. Top each with crushed pineapple. Pour orange juice over chops. Cover and bake for 1 hour.

VEAL PARMESAN

Preheat oven to 350° F.   SERVES 4

(1 serving=3 meat exchanges, 1½ fat exchanges, and 2
vegetable exchanges)

8 ounces veal cutlet
1 teaspoon salt
Dash pepper
2 cups chopped onion
4 teaspoons butter
2 cups Tomato Sauce*

½ teaspoon basil
½ teaspoon oregano
3 ounces mozzarella cheese
3 tablespoons grated Parmesan
   cheese

Pound veal until thin. Season with salt and pepper. Sauté onion
and veal in butter until brown. Place in baking dish. Pour over
tomato sauce. Sprinkle with basil and oregano. Top with
cheeses. Cover and bake for 45 minutes.

VEAL STEW

SERVES 4 TO 6

(1 ounce veal=1 meat exchange)
(½ cup onion=1 vegetable exchange)
(1 potato=1 bread exchange)

4 cups water
2 pounds veal stew meat
½ cup sliced onion
¼ cup sliced carrot
1 bay leaf
3 peppercorns
2 teaspoons salt
1 teaspoon MSG

1 small clove garlic
¼ teaspoon oregano
1 cup sliced mushrooms
2 tablespoons lemon juice
2 tablespoons Tomato Sauce*
1 tablespoon chopped parsley
3 cups small white onions, boiled
6 small new potatoes, boiled

Bring water to a boil. Add veal, onion, carrot, bay leaf, peppercorns, salt, MSG, garlic, and oregano. Simmer until meat is tender. Skim off surface scum as it appears. Remove bay leaf and peppercorns. Add mushrooms, lemon juice, and tomato sauce and cook 20 minutes. Sprinkle with parsley. Serve with onions and potatoes.

BAKED HERB CHICKEN

Preheat oven to 325° F.   SERVES 4

(1 ounce=1 meat exchange)

1 frying chicken, quartered
1 cup chicken bouillon
1 teaspoon grated lemon rind

2 tablespoons lemon juice
¼ teaspoon basil
¼ teaspoon oregano

Place chicken in baking dish. Combine remaining ingredients and pour over chicken. Cover and bake for 1¼ hours. Remove cover for last 30 minutes.

BARBECUED CHICKEN*
•
BOILED CHICKEN

SERVES 6 TO 8

(1 ounce=1 meat exchange)

1 4-to-5 pound chicken, whole or cut up	1 slice onion
	1 sprig parsley
1 quart hot water	1 carrot
1 rib celery	1 tablespoon salt

Place chicken in kettle. Add remaining ingredients and bring to the boiling point. Cover and simmer over low heat until tender, 1½ to 2½ hours. Let the chicken cool in the liquid. The stock may be used for soup. The stock need not be counted as an exchange.

CHINESE CHICKEN

Preheat oven to 350° F.

SERVES 4

(1 ounce=1 meat exchange)

1 2½-to-3 pound chicken	1 teaspoon ginger
¾ cup water	1 clove garlic, crushed
½ cup soy sauce	
2½ teaspoons granulated sugar substitute (substitute for ½ cup sugar)	

Place chicken in baking dish. Combine remaining ingredients and pour over chicken. Marinate several hours, turning occasionally. Cover and bake for 1 hour.

CHICKEN CHOW MEIN

SERVES 4

(1 serving=2 meat exchanges, 2 vegetable exchanges, and 1 bread exchange)

1 cup finely shredded cooked chicken
4 cups canned mixed Chinese vegetables, drained
1 cup chicken bouillon
1 tablespoon cornstarch

¼ teaspoon granulated sugar substitute (substitute for 1 tablespoon sugar)
1 tablespoon soy sauce
2 tablespoons water
2 cups chow mein noodles

Combine chicken, vegetables, and bouillon and bring to a boil. Combine cornstarch, sweetener, soy sauce, and water. Add to chicken and vegetables and cook until thickened, stirring constantly. Serve over noodles.

OVEN-FRIED CHICKEN

Preheat oven to 400° F.

SERVES 4

(1 ounce chicken=1 meat exchange)

1 2½-to-3-pound chicken, cut up
2 ounces coating mix (below)

Moisten chicken and roll in coating mix or shake in a paper or plastic bag. Arrange chicken in a baking dish and bake for 45 minutes.

A good rule to follow in purchasing any fowl is to allow ½ pound per average serving.

COATING FOR OVEN-FRIED CHICKEN

MAKES 2½ CUPS

(need not be counted as an exchange)

2 cups bread crumbs	1 teaspoon onion salt
1½ teaspoons salt	¼ teaspoon pepper
1½ teaspoons paprika	1 teaspoon poultry seasoning
1 teaspoon celery salt	¼ cup vegetable oil

Blend all ingredients together with fork or pastry blender. Store unrefrigerated in a tightly covered container.

CORNISH HENS

Preheat oven to 450° F.   SERVES 4

(1 ounce hen=1 meat exchange)

4 Cornish hens	1 tart apple, sliced
Salt and pepper to taste	1 cup unsweetened apple juice

Season hens with salt and pepper. Put a few slices of apple in the cavity of each. Place in roasting pan and pour apple juice over hens. Baste several times during cooking with apple juice and drippings. Roast uncovered for 10 minutes. Lower heat to 350° and roast 25 minutes longer.

CRISP ROAST DUCKLING

Preheat oven to 425° F.   SERVES 4

(1 ounce=1 meat exchange and 1 fat exchange)

1 5-pound duckling	**1 teaspoon caraway seeds**
2 teaspoons salt	**½ cup water**

Salt cavity of duck with 1 teaspoon salt and sprinkle remaining salt and caraway seeds on outside of duck. Place on a rack in a roasting pan with ½ cup water. Cover and roast for 1½ hours. At ½ hour intervals, remove cover and pierce skin of entire duck to allow fat to exude. Be sure to cut skin between legs and body. Remove cover and drain fat from the pan (this may be done with a bulb baster). Reduce oven temperature to 325° and roast uncovered for 2 more hours. Continue to pierce skin and turn duck at ½ hour intervals. Raise heat to 350°, turn duck breast side up and roast ½ hour longer. For additional crispness, allow duck to remain in oven for ½ hour with heat turned off.

ROAST GOOSE WITH SAUERKRAUT

Preheat oven to 325° F.   SERVES 8 TO 10

(1 ounce goose=1 meat exchange and 1 fat exchange)
(1 cup stuffing=1¼ vegetable exchanges, ¼ bread exchange, and ½ fruit exchange)

4 pounds sauerkraut	1 tablespoon caraway seeds
2 cups finely chopped onion	Salt and freshly ground pepper to
2 cups finely chopped apple	taste
1 cup grated potato	1 8-to-10-pound goose
½ teaspoon salt	

Drain sauerkraut. Wash it under cold running water, then soak it in cold water for 15 minutes. Squeeze the sauerkraut dry and put it into a large mixing bowl. Add onion, apple, potato, ½ teaspoon salt, caraway seeds, and a few grindings of pepper.

Wash the goose inside and out with cold running water. Pat it dry with paper towels. Sprinkle the cavity generously with salt and a few grindings of pepper. Fill with sauerkraut stuffing. Sew the openings with a needle and thread and tie the legs. Place the goose, breast side up, on a rack in a roasting pan. Roast for 25 minutes per pound. Occasionally remove fat from the pan with bulb baster. Let the goose rest on a platter for 15 to 20 minutes before carving.

ROAST TURKEY*

GAME

Hunting season need not present any problems when you are preparing meals for your diabetic child. Just remember that 1 ounce of bear, deer, buffalo, muskrat, raccoon, squirrel, rabbit, pheasant, wild duck, or partridge=1 meat exchange and 1 fat exchange.

I am unable to give you any favorite recipes for cooking game. Many wild creatures have been temporary residents in my home, but they were all very much alive and I kept my distance. My children, most certainly, would have deserted me had I ever served them a rabbit stew or a fried squirrel. My knowledge, therefore, is limited to a few basic facts.

All large game, some small game, and most game birds must hang before they are ready to eat, just as beef must be hung until it is tender. After hanging, large game can be cooked like similar cuts of meat, and small game and game birds like poultry. Birds should be plucked and animals skinned before hanging in a cool airy place for the following lengths of time:

bear	—	5 days
deer	—	2 to 4 weeks
grouse	—	2 weeks
partridge	—	4 days
pheasant	—	4 days
raccoon	—	2 days
wild duck	—	1 week
wild goose	—	1 week
woodcock	—	4 days

FISH

Fish is a good food to feed to your diabetic child, because it is one of the most nourishing of foods. Very few foods can equal fish in nutritive value. It is rich in proteins, vitamins, and minerals, and it is also very rich in iodine.

Like fruits and vegetables, fish are most economical to buy when in season. A great many varieties are quick-frozen as soon as caught and may be purchased in this way whether in or out of season.

When purchasing fish allow ⅓ pound per person for steaks and fillets, and 1 pound per person for whole fish. Select fish with bright, clear, bulging eyes; reddish-pink gills; scales that adhere tightly to the skin; firm and elastic flesh that springs back when pressed and that is free from objectionable odors. Fish should be stored in the refrigerator in a tightly covered container or wrapped in waterproof paper. This will keep the odor of the fish from penetrating other foods in the refrigerator.

The most common error made in cooking fish is to cook it too long. Overcooking draws out most of the natural juices and causes the flesh to shrink and become dried out. A good rule to follow in cooking fish is to measure it at its thickest point, in depth, and cook it for 10 minutes per inch. This applies to steaks, fillets, and whole fish. It applies to fish that is baked, broiled, fried, or poached. In baking, use a preheated 450° F. oven.

BAKED FISH

Preheat oven to 450° F.   SERVES 6

(1 ounce fish=1 meat exchange)
(3 tablespoons sauce=⅓ vegetable exchange)

2 pounds fish, in season	1 tablespoon minced onion
3 tablespoons lemon juice	2 tablespoons chopped fresh
Salt and pepper to taste	parsley
1 cup Tomato Sauce*	1 tablespoon Parmesan cheese
½ teaspoon oregano	

Dip fish in 2 tablespoons lemon juice. Season with salt and pepper. Place in a greased shallow baking dish. Bake uncovered for 15 minutes. Remove from oven and drain off liquid. Reduce heat to 375°. Combine remaining lemon juice, tomato sauce, oregano, and onion. Bring to a boil and cook 2 minutes. Pour over fish. Sprinkle with parsley and cheese. Bake 15 minutes longer.

BROILED FISH

Preheat broiler   SERVES 6

(1 ounce fish=1 meat exchange)

2 pounds fish fillets, in season	2 tablespoons chopped fresh
Salt and pepper to taste	parsley
2 tablespoons lemon juice	

Place fish, skin side up, on aluminum foil and crimp sides to form a boat shape. Sprinkle fish with salt, pepper, lemon juice, and parsley. Broil 3 inches from the flame for 10 minutes. Carefully turn and broil 5 minutes longer.

FISH CAKES

Preheat oven to 450° F. SERVES 4

(1 fish cake=2 meat exchanges and ½ bread exchange)

2 cups shredded cooked fish	½ teaspoon salt
2 cups seasoned mashed potatoes	1 egg, beaten
¼ teaspoon pepper	½ cup chopped onion

Mix all ingredients. Shape into 8 cakes. Bake for 15 minutes. To brown cakes, place them under broiler until golden brown.

For a hearty meal on a cold winter day, try:

FISH CHOWDER

SERVES 4

(1 serving=2 meat exchanges, 1 bread exchange, 1 milk exchange, ¼ vegetable exchange, and 1 fat exchange)

8 ounces haddock	4 cups skim milk
1 medium onion, chopped	1 teaspoon salt
4 teaspoons butter	¼ teaspoon pepper
4 potatoes, sliced	Chopped fresh parsley
½ cup water	

Cook fish in lightly salted water for 15 minutes or until tender. Brown onion in butter. Add potatoes and water. Cover and cook until potatoes are tender. Add milk, salt, and pepper. Remove skin and bones from fish. Dice and add to milk mixture. Reheat and serve garnished with parsley.

Whenever you increase a recipe, be sure to increase all the ingredients proportionately.

POACHED FISH

SERVES 6

(1 ounce fish=1 meat exchange)

3 quarts water	1 carrot
1 teaspoon salt	1 celery rib
2 tablespoons lemon juice	2 pounds fish fillets
3 peppercorns	Paprika
1 bay leaf	Lemon wedges
¼ cup sliced onion	

Combine all ingredients except fillets and bring to a boil. Cook over low heat for 20 minutes. Place fish in mixture and simmer 10 minutes or until tender. Serve garnished with paprika and lemon wedges.

Adventuresome teenagers may enjoy serving this appetizer to their friends:

SWEDISH SALMON

SERVES 12 TO 15

(1 ounce fish=1 meat exchange)

3 pounds fresh salmon fillets
1 bunch fresh dill
¼ cup salt
2 tablespoons peppercorns,
  crushed

1 teaspoon granulated sugar
  substitute (substitute for ¼ cup
  sugar)
Lemon wedges

Place half of the fish, skin side down, in a glass baking dish. Wash and dry dill and place it on the fish. Combine salt, pepper, and sweetener. Sprinkle this mixture evenly over the dill. Top with the other half of the fish, skin side up. Cover with aluminum foil. Refrigerate 48 hours, turning the fish every 12 hours. It may be marinated up to 3 days. Remove the salmon from the marinade, scrape away the dill and seasonings. Slice the salmon thinly on the diagonal and detach from the skin. Serve with lemon wedges.

TUNA BURGERS

SERVES 4

(1 serving=1 meat exchange and 2 bread exchanges)

1 7-ounce can water-packed tuna
½ 10½-ounce can condensed
  cream of chicken soup
Juice of 1 lemon
¼ cup chopped celery

2 tablespoons chopped onion
1 tablespoon parsley
Pepper to taste
4 toasted buns, split

Combine all ingredients except buns and cook over a low flame for 5 minutes. Serve on toasted buns.

CASSEROLES

Casseroles are an easy, quick way to prepare meals and they are usually inexpensive. They can be prepared in advance and stored in the refrigerator until you are ready to pop them into the oven. They can be frozen when either partially or fully cooked. To bake frozen food that is partially cooked, use the temperature given in the recipe and add ½ hour to the cooking time. To bake frozen foods that are fully cooked use the time and temperature given in the recipe. Do not thaw before cooking.

Casserole cooking is generally a form of oven cooking, but some casseroles may be prepared on top of the stove. Most casseroles are very hearty, and often a salad, beverage, and simple dessert are all that is needed to complete the meal.

BEEF NOODLE CASSEROLE

Preheat oven to 325° F.   SERVES 6

(1 serving=2 meat exchanges, 1 fat exchange, 2 vegetable exchanges, and 1 bread exchange)

Shaker of salt
¾ pound lean ground beef
1 cup chopped onion
1 cup sliced mushrooms

Salt and pepper to taste
3 cups cooked fine noodles
1 28-ounce can seasoned tomatoes

Sprinkle salt in the bottom of skillet. Add meat and brown over low flame. Add onion and mushrooms and sauté until tender. Season to taste with salt and pepper. Put beef mixture in the bottom of a lightly greased casserole; top with noodles; pour tomatoes over all. Bake 30 minutes.

CHILI

SERVES 6

(1 serving=2⅓ vegetable exchanges, 2 meat exchanges, 1 fat exchange, and 1⅓ bread exchanges)

1 28-ounce can tomatoes
1 6-ounce can tomato paste
Salt and pepper to taste
¾ pound lean ground beef
1 cup chopped onion

1 cup chopped green pepper
1 cup chopped celery
1 16-ounce can kidney beans
1 tablespoon chili powder

Combine tomatoes and tomato paste. Season with salt and pepper and simmer for 20 minutes. Sprinkle skillet with salt, add meat, and brown over low heat. Add onion, green pepper, and celery and sauté until tender. Combine meat mixture with tomatoes and simmer for 2 hours. Add kidney beans. Season with chili powder and salt to taste. Simmer 30 minutes.

HOT DOG CASSEROLE

SERVES 6

(1 serving=1 meat exchange, 1½ fat exchanges, 1 vegetable exchange, and 1 bread exchange)

1 cup chopped onion	Dash pepper
1 tablespoon oil	1 teaspoon parsley
1 cup chopped green pepper	½ teaspoon oregano
1 cup Tomato Sauce*	6 hot dogs, cut in quarters
¼ teaspoon salt	3 cups cooked rice

Sauté onions in oil until transparent. Add green pepper and cook until soft. Add tomato sauce and seasonings. Cook for 15 minutes. Add hot dogs and cook 5 minutes more. Serve over cooked rice.

LASAGNE

Preheat oven to 350° F.

SERVES 6

(1 serving=3 meat exchanges, 1½ vegetable exchanges, 1½ fat exchanges, and 1 bread exchange)

6 pieces of lasagne	¼ teaspoon salt
Shaker of salt	Dash pepper
½ pound lean ground beef	¼ teaspoon oregano
½ cup chopped celery	½ pound mozzarella cheese,
½ cup chopped onion	thinly sliced
1 clove garlic, minced	3 tablespoons grated Parmesan
1 28-ounce can tomatoes	cheese
1 6-ounce can tomato paste	

Cook lasagne according to package directions. Drain and rinse. Sprinkle skillet with salt and brown beef over low heat. Add celery, onion, and garlic and cook until tender. Add tomatoes, tomato paste, and seasonings. Simmer 1½ hours. In a greased casserole, arrange alternate layers of lasagne, sauce, and mozzarella, ending with sauce. Sprinkle with Parmesan. Bake for 30 minutes.

MACARONI AND CHEESE

Preheat oven to 325° F.   SERVES 6

(1 serving=1 bread exchange, ½ vegetable exchange, 1 fat exchange, and 1 meat exchange)

3 cups cooked elbow macaroni
1½ cups Tomato Sauce*
6 ounces sharp cheese, grated

Combine all ingredients. Bake in a lightly greased casserole for 30 minutes.

NOODLES ROMANOFF

Preheat oven to 350° F.   SERVES 6

(1 serving=1 bread exchange, 1⅓ fat exchanges, and ⅔ meat exchange)

3 cups cooked medium noodles   **3 tablespoons chives**
1 cup cottage cheese   **1 teaspoon salt**
1 cup sour cream   **1 tablespoon Worcestershire sauce**
2 cloves garlic, minced

Combine all ingredients and bake in lightly greased casserole for 30 minutes.

SHEPHERD'S PIE*
●
SLOPPY HOT DOGS

Preheat oven to 350° F.   SERVES 4

(1 serving=1 meat exchange, ⅔ vegetable exchange, 1 fat exchange, and 2 bread exchanges)

4 hot dogs, sliced	½ cup chopped green pepper
1 cup baked beans	⅓ cup Tomato Sauce*
½ cup chopped onion	2 hot dog rolls, toasted

Combine all ingredients except rolls and bake in lightly greased covered casserole for 30 minutes. Serve on half a hot dog roll.

SPANISH RICE

Preheat oven to 350° F.   SERVES 4

(1 serving=2 vegetable exchanges, 1 fat exchange, and 1 bread exchange)

1 clove garlic, minced	1 cup rice
4 teaspoons olive oil	2 tablespoons chopped fresh
1 cup chopped onion	parsley
1 cup chopped green pepper	1 cup beef bouillon
2 cups chopped tomatoes	Salt and pepper to taste

Brown garlic in oil. Add onion, green pepper, and tomatoes and sauté until soft. Add rice and parsley and cook until rice is brown. Add bouillon. Season with salt and pepper. Bake in a covered casserole for 35 minutes.

BAKED TUNA WITH NOODLES

Preheat oven to 350° F.   SERVES 4

(1 serving=1 meat exchange, ½ milk exchange, and 1½ bread exchanges)

1 7-ounce can water-packed tuna	1 tablespoon grated onion
1 10½-ounce can condensed cream of celery soup	¼ teaspoon salt
	3 tablespoons chopped pimiento
¾ cup milk	2 cups cooked fine noodles
1 tablespoon lemon juice	2 tablespoons bread crumbs

Combine all ingredients except bread crumbs. Pour into baking dish. Top with crumbs. Bake for 30 minutes.

VEGETABLES

Vegetables are at their best when they are steamed over boiling water or cooked in a small amount of boiling water. If you boil vegetables in a large amount of water for too long a period of time, you will also boil away all of the minerals and vitamins. We would do well to take a lesson from the Chinese, and I don't mean on how to iron shirts. They were skilled in the culinary arts long before the Western Hemisphere was even envisioned. They always cook their vegetables until they are al dente, or just a bit underdone.

Always try to use those vegetables that are in season. They are less expensive and have more flavor. There is a chart in Appendix E indicating when each of the vegetables is at the peak of its growth.

Your diabetic child will benefit from a variety of different kinds of vegetables. Try to help him to develop a taste for as many different vegetables as possible. Each one is rich in a different source of minerals and vitamins. Eating a variety of different foods will always be the key to good health for your diabetic child.

ARTICHOKES WITH MOCK HOLLANDAISE

(1 artichoke=1 vegetable exchange)

Trim the base of the artichoke flush and flat. Remove small bottom leaves and any bruised outer leaves. Place artichokes in boiling salted water and boil uncovered until tender, about 45 minutes. Remove them from the cooking water with tongs. Place them upside down on a rack or in a colander to drain. Serve with mock hollandaise (below).

MOCK HOLLANDAISE

MAKES ⅔ CUP

(2 tablespoons need not be counted as an exchange)

½ cup skim milk
2 tablespoons flour
½ teaspoon salt

½ teaspoon dry mustard
3 tablespoons lemon juice

Combine milk, flour, salt, and dry mustard. Cook, stirring constantly, until thickened. Continue to stir and slowly add lemon juice. Store in a covered container.

BUTTERED ASPARAGUS

(½ cup asparagus=1 vegetable exchange)
(1 teaspoon butter=1 fat exchange)

Cut off the tough end of the asparagus, so that all the spears are about the same length. Asparagus spears may be peeled. Peeling helps to retain the green color. Place the asparagus in boiling salted water and boil uncovered for 8 to 10 minutes or steam over boiling water until tender. Drain and serve with melted butter or lemon butter.

The flavor of all vegetables is enhanced by the addition of melted butter. This is the ideal place for the diabetic to use the fat exchanges. For this reason, I have used as little fat as possible with the other five exchanges.

GREEN BEANS NIÇOISE

SERVES 6

(½ cup=1 vegetable exchange)

1 pound string beans
3 tomatoes, sliced
2 onions, sliced
3 green peppers, quartered

Salt and pepper to taste
1 bay leaf
6 sprigs parsley

Break string beans into 2-inch pieces. Layer vegetables in a heavy casserole. Sprinkle with salt and pepper. Add bay leaf and parsley and cook over the lowest possible heat until tender. This will take several hours.

BEETS WITH HORSERADISH

SERVES 4

(1 serving=1 vegetable exchange and ¼ fruit exchange)

2 cups sliced cooked beets
1 small apple, peeled, cored, and
   diced
½ cup vinegar
¼ teaspoon granulated sugar
   substitute (substitute for 1
   tablespoon sugar)

½ teaspoon salt
1 teaspoon caraway seeds
2 teaspoons prepared horseradish

Combine beets and apple. Simmer vinegar, sweetener, and salt over low heat for 5 minutes. Add caraway seeds and horseradish. Pour over beets and apple. Cool to room temperature. Cover and refrigerate at least 12 hours.

GLAZED BEETS

SERVES 6

(1 serving=1 vegetable exchange and 1 fat exchange)

2 tablespoons butter
2 teaspoons cornstarch
¼ teaspoon salt
2½ teaspoons granulated sugar substitute (substitute for ½ cup sugar)

1 teaspoon vinegar
2 teaspoons grated orange rind
½ cup orange juice
3 cups sliced cooked beets

Melt butter and add cornstarch. Stir until well blended. Add salt, sweetener, vinegar, orange rind, and orange juice. Cook over low heat, stirring constantly, until the sauce is thickened. Add beets and simmer 10 minutes.

BRUSSELS SPROUTS WITH PIMIENTO*
●
BRUSSELS SPROUTS IN CHICKEN STOCK

SERVES 6

(1 serving=1 vegetable exchange and 1 fat exchange)

3 cups brussels sprouts
2 tablespoons butter
1 medium onion, thinly sliced
⅓ cup chicken bouillon

1 teaspoon chopped fresh parsley
1 teaspoon chopped chives
Salt and pepper to taste

Cook brussels sprouts in a little boiling water for 5 minutes. Drain. Melt butter in saucepan and cook onion in it until soft. Add bouillon and brussels sprouts. Simmer for 5 minutes. Sprinkle with parsley and chives and season with salt and pepper.

BRAISED CABBAGE

Preheat oven to 300° F.   SERVES 4

(1 serving=1½ vegetable exchanges and 1½ fat exchanges)

1 1-pound head cabbage	1 bay leaf
6 slices bacon	1 tablespoon chopped fresh
1 carrot, sliced	parsley
1 small onion, sliced	½ teaspoon thyme
2 cloves	1¼ cups beef bouillon

Cut cabbage in quarters and cook in boiling salted water until tender. Drain well. Place 3 slices of bacon in the bottom of a casserole. Add cabbage, carrot, onion, cloves, bay leaf, parsley, thyme, and bouillon. Top with remaining bacon. Bake 2 hours.

SWEET AND SOUR RED CABBAGE

SERVES 6

(1 serving=1 vegetable exchange, ⅔ fruit exchange, and ½ fat exchange)

1 1-pound head red cabbage	1 tablespoon cider vinegar
1 tablespoon butter	⅔ cup unsweetened apple juice
2 small onions, sliced	2 small tart apples
¼ teaspoon granulated brown sugar substitute (substitute for 1 tablespoon brown sugar)	

Shred cabbage, wash, and drain well. Melt butter and sauté onions until soft. Stir in sweetener and vinegar. Add cabbage and apple juice. Simmer for 1 hour. Peel and core apples and cut into eighths. Stir into cabbage. Season to taste and continue cooking for 1 hour.

BAKED CARROTS

Preheat oven to 325° F.   SERVES 6

(1 serving=1 vegetable exchange and 1 fat exchange)

3 cups carrots, pared and cut in quarters	⅛ teaspoon pepper
½ teaspoon salt	2 tablespoons butter

Place carrots in a buttered casserole. Sprinkle with salt and pepper and dot with butter. Cover and bake for 1¼ hours.

Carrots taste extra sweet when cooked this way because all of the flavor is retained.

All frozen vegetables may be cooked in the oven without the addition of any liquid. It is an excellent way to preserve the minerals and vitamins.

ORANGE CARROTS

SERVES 6

(1 serving=1 vegetable exchange, 1 fat exchange, and ⅓ fruit exchange)

3 cups sliced cooked carrots
1 cup mandarin oranges
2 tablespoons butter

Combine all ingredients and cook over low heat for 5 minutes.

CAULIFLOWER AU GRATIN

SERVES 6

(½ cup=1 vegetable exchange, 1 fat exchange, and 1 meat exchange)

1 medium head cauliflower, separated into flowerets
Salt and pepper to taste
6 ounces sharp Cheddar cheese, shredded

Boil cauliflower until just tender. Drain. Sprinkle with salt and pepper. Add cheese and heat slowly until cheese melts.

EGGPLANT PROVENÇALE

Preheat oven to 350° F.   SERVES 6

(½ cup=1 vegetable exchange)

1 eggplant, peeled and cut in
  ¼-inch slices
1 medium onion, sliced
4 tomatoes, peeled and quartered
1 green pepper, chopped

Salt and pepper to taste
Chopped fresh parsley
3 tablespoons grated Parmesan
  cheese

Place a layer of eggplant in a greased baking dish. Top with a layer of onion, tomato, and green pepper. Sprinkle with salt and pepper. Alternate layers of the vegetables. Top with chopped parsley and Parmesan. Bake for 45 minutes.

EGGPLANT RELISH

Preheat oven to 500° F.   SERVES 6

(½ cup=1 vegetable exchange)

1 large eggplant
3 large green peppers
1 teaspoon salt

½ teaspoon finely chopped garlic
2 tablespoons finely chopped fresh
  parsley

Place eggplant and green peppers on a rack in a baking pan. Bake green peppers for 25 minutes. Bake eggplant for 40 minutes. Wrap eggplant in a damp towel. Allow vegetables to cool. Peel green peppers, remove the seeds and membranes, and chop very fine. Peel the eggplant, chop it very fine, and squeeze out excess moisture. Combine peppers and eggplant. Season with salt and stir in the garlic. Chill and garnish with parsley.

OKRA AND TOMATOES

SERVES 4

(1 cup=2 vegetable exchanges)

1 package frozen okra
½ cup chopped onion
2 cups peeled cubed tomatoes

2 teaspoons salt
Dash pepper

Cut okra in ½-inch pieces. Combine with remaining ingredients. Cook 10 to 15 minutes.

BAKED STUFFED ONIONS

Preheat oven to 375° F.   SERVES 6

(1 stuffed onion cup=1 vegetable exchange, 1 fat exchange, and ¼ bread exchange)

3 large onions
Paprika
2 tablespoons butter
1 tablespoon cornstarch
¾ cup canned peas, with 1 cup
   liquid drained from peas

2 tablespoons chopped pimiento
¼ teaspoon salt
¼ teaspoon Worcestershire sauce

Peel onions and cut them in half, crosswise. Cut out enough of the inside to leave a shell ¾ inch thick. Sprinkle onion cups with paprika. Bake in a covered casserole for 20 minutes. Chop enough onion centers to make ¼ cup. Sauté in butter until tender. Add cornstarch and stir until well blended. Add liquid from peas and cook over low heat, stirring constantly, until the sauce is thickened. Add peas, pimiento, salt, and Worcestershire. Fill onion cups with mixture. Cover and bake for 15 minutes.

GLAZED ONIONS*
●
BRAISED PEAS

SERVES 6

(1 serving=1 bread exchange and 1 fat exchange)

1 head Boston lettuce
3 cups shelled fresh green peas
6 sprigs parsley, tied
½ cup water
½ teaspoon salt

⅛ teaspoon granulated sugar substitute (substitute for 1 teaspoon sugar)
2 tablespoons butter

Wash lettuce, remove any wilted outer leaves, and cut into 6 wedges. Bring lettuce, peas, parsley, water, salt, and sweetener to a boil. Cover, reduce heat, and simmer for about 15 minutes. The liquid should be cooked away. Remove parsley and stir in butter.

APPLE CHEESE POTATOES

Preheat oven to 375° F.

SERVES 4

(1 serving=1 bread exchange, ½ meat exchange, ¼ fat exchange, and ½ fruit exchange)

4 small potatoes
Salt and pepper to taste

6 tablespoons Parmesan cheese
⅔ cup unsweetened apple juice

Cut potatoes in slices and put half in a lightly greased baking dish. Sprinkle with salt, pepper, and half the cheese. Repeat. Add the apple juice. Cover and bake for 1½ hours.

POTATO-BACON-ONION BAKE

Preheat oven to 400° F. SERVES 6

(1 serving=1 bread exchange and 1 fat exchange)

3 cups cubed cooked potatoes
Salt and pepper to taste
6 slices bacon, chopped

½ cup thinly sliced onion
½ cup milk

Lightly grease baking dish. Place half the potatoes in the bottom of the dish. Season with salt and pepper. Cover with bacon and onion. Top with remaining potatoes. Pour milk over top. Cover and bake for 30 minutes. Remove the cover and bake 15 minutes longer.

PARSLEYED POTATOES

SERVES 6

(1 serving=1 bread exchange and 1 fat exchange)

12 new small potatoes
2 tablespoons butter
3 tablespoons chopped fresh parsley

Cook potatoes in boiling, salted water for 20 minutes. Drain and peel. Melt butter in saucepan. Add parsley and potatoes. Shake gently to cover potatoes with butter and parsley.

POTATOES WITH SOUR CREAM

Preheat oven to 350° F.   SERVES 6

(1 serving=1 bread exchange and ½ fat exchange)

3 cups mashed potatoes   ¼ teaspoon pepper
6 tablespoons sour cream   3 tablespoons chopped chives
1 teaspoon salt   Paprika

Combine all ingredients except paprika. Put into a lightly greased baking dish and sprinkle with paprika. Bake 30 minutes.

SWEET POTATOES ON PINEAPPLE RINGS

Preheat oven to 400° F.   SERVES 6

(1 serving=1 bread exchange, 1 fat exchange, and 1 fruit exchange)

1½ cups mashed cooked sweet   ¼ teaspoon cinnamon
   potatoes   ¼ teaspoon nutmeg
2 tablespoons butter, melted   6 slices water-packed pineapple
2½ teaspoons granulated brown
   sugar substitute (substitute for
   ½ cup brown sugar)

Mix potatoes, butter, sweetener, cinnamon, and nutmeg. Place in mounds on pineapple rings and bake for 10 minutes.

BAKED RUTABAGAS

Preheat oven to 375° F.   SERVES 6

(½ cup=1 vegetable exchange and 1 fat exchange)

6 rutabagas   2 tablespoons butter
2 tablespoons lemon juice
2 tablespoons chopped fresh
    parsley

Wash rutabagas and bake them unpeeled for 1½ hours. Cut them in half and sprinkle them with lemon juice and chopped parsley. Serve 1 teaspoon of butter with each ½ cup serving.

SNAPS

SERVES 4

(1 serving=2 vegetable exchanges)

2 cups cooked green beans   1 tomato, chopped
1 cup chopped purple Italian   Salt and pepper to taste
    onion

Mix beans, onion, and tomatoes. Season with salt and pepper. Serve cold.

Snaps are a great summer favorite in the South. Platters of sliced onions and tomatoes are served along with green beans, and everyone makes his own at the table.

SUMMER SQUASH AU GRATIN

SERVES 4

(1 serving=1 vegetable exchange, 1 meat exchange, and 2 fat exchanges)

2 cups cubed summer squash   4 teaspoons butter
4 teaspoons chopped pimiento   4 ounces sharp cheese, shredded

Cook the squash in boiling salted water for 20 minutes or until tender. Drain and add remaining ingredients. Heat slowly until cheese melts.

BAKED TOMATOES

Preheat oven to 425° F.

(1 tomato=1 vegetable exchange)

Use small tomatoes of even size and leave them whole. Slash the tops in a cross and arrange them in a well-greased baking dish or tin. Bake until the tops split and are browned.

GRILLED TOMATOES

(1 tomato=1 vegetable exchange and 1 fat exchange)

Cut small tomatoes in half. Season with salt and pepper. Top each half with a sprinkling of bread crumbs and ½ teaspoon butter. Broil until the crumbs are brown and the skin is wrinkled.

TOMATOES AND ONIONS

Preheat oven to 425° F.   SERVES 6

(1 serving=1½ vegetable exchanges, ⅓ meat exchange, and ½ bread exchange)

1 pound onions
Salt and pepper to taste
½ teaspoon basil
2 pounds tomatoes

1 cup soft bread crumbs
6 tablespoons grated Parmesan cheese

Peel and slice onions and boil in salted water for 20 minutes. Drain well and season with salt, pepper, and basil. Put half in the bottom of a greased casserole. Peel and slice tomatoes and put half on top of the onions. Sprinkle with half the bread crumbs and cheese. Repeat. Bake for 20 minutes.

WHITE TURNIPS

SERVES 6

(½ cup=1 vegetable exchange and 1 fat exchange)

12 small white turnips, peeled   2 tablespoons butter
1 cup chicken bouillon
¼ teaspoon granulated sugar
    substitute (substitute for 2
    teaspoons sugar)

Cut turnips into ¼-inch slices and parboil in salted water for 5 minutes. Drain the water and rinse turnips in cold water. Cover with chicken bouillon, add sweetener, and cook for 15 minutes. Drain. Melt butter and pour over turnips.

WINTER SQUASH*
●
ZUCCHINI

SERVES 4

(1 serving=1 vegetable exchange and 1 fat exchange)

2 cups ½-inch zucchini squares   4 teaspoons lemon juice
4 teaspoons butter   1 cup chopped fresh parsley
4 teaspoons minced onion

Cook zucchini in a small amount of boiling, salted water until just tender. Drain. Combine butter, onion, and lemon juice. Heat until butter is melted. Pour over squash. Add parsley and mix thoroughly.

SALADS

Salads are an interesting way to use most of the exchanges. Fruits, vegetables, meat, fish, and poultry are easily combined to make for whole meals or accompaniments to entrées. Always serve salads that are crisp and well chilled. Never serve them if they are left over or wilted. Most children enjoy fruit salads and they are a special treat when accompanied by a sherbet. Salads give you lots of opportunities to use your imagination and creativity.

To unmold a molded salad with ease, grease the mold with mayonnaise before pouring the salad into it. When you are ready to unmold the salad, dip the mold into warm water, not hot, to the depth of the gelatin. Loosen around the edges of the mold with the tip of a sharp knife. If salad does not unmold readily, repeat the procedure. If you do not have a salad mold, use a glass or Pyrex bowl lined with plastic wrap.

MOLDED BEEF SALAD

SERVES 4

(1 serving=2 meat exchanges and 1 fat exchange)

1 envelope unflavored gelatin	1 teaspoon salt
1 cup water	1 cup diced cooked beef
1 cup beef bouillon	½ cup diced apple
1 tablespoon grated onion	2 tablespoons chopped celery
1 tablespoon vinegar	Lettuce leaves

Soak gelatin in ¼ cup cold water. Bring bouillon to a boil and pour over gelatin. Stir until dissolved. Add remaining ¾ cup water, onion, vinegar, and salt. Chill until slightly thickened. Fold in beef, apple, and celery. Chill until firm. Serve on a bed of lettuce.

CARROT AND RAISIN SALAD

SERVES 4

(1 serving=1 vegetable exchange, 1 fat exchange, and ½ fruit exchange)

1 cup water	2 teaspoons lemon juice
1 teaspoon vinegar	¼ teaspoon granulated sugar
4 tablespoons raisins	substitute (substitute for 2½
2 cups grated carrots	teaspoons sugar)
4 teaspoons mayonnaise	

Combine water, vinegar, and raisins. Bring to a boil, turn off heat, and allow raisins to soak for 5 minutes. Drain raisins and combine with remaining ingredients. Chill.

COLESLAW

SERVES 8

(1 serving=1 vegetable exchange)

3 cups shredded cabbage
½ cup chopped green pepper
½ cup grated onion

½ cup grated carrot
Yogurt Salad Dressing*

Combine all ingredients and chill.

MOLDED GREEN SALAD

SERVES 6

(1 serving=1 vegetable exchange)

1 envelope unflavored gelatin
1¾ cups water
¼ teaspoon granulated sugar
  substitute (substitute for 1
  tablespoon sugar)
1 teaspoon salt
¼ cup vinegar

1 tablespoon lemon juice
¼ cup chopped scallions
1 cup shredded raw spinach
1 cup chopped celery
1 cup shredded carrots
Salad greens

Soak gelatin in ¼ cup cold water. Add ½ cup boiling water and stir until dissolved. Add sweetener and salt. Stir in remaining cup of water, vinegar, and lemon juice. Chill mixture to unbeaten egg white consistency. Fold in vegetables. Pour into mold and chill until firm. Unmold on serving dish and garnish with salad greens.

Serve with 2 tablespoons low-fat cottage cheese. Add ½ meat exchange.

TOSSED GREEN SALAD

(need not be counted as an exchange)

Use young, fresh, unblemished greens. Wash thoroughly and dry. Break greens into bite-size pieces using your fingers. The best salad bowl is a wooden bowl and it should be used exclusively for tossing the salad. Rub it with a cut clove of garlic. Add the salad dressing at the last possible minute and toss until every green leaf glistens. Season with freshly ground pepper and salt.

Suggested greens: romaine, simpson, Boston, and iceberg lettuce; escarole, chicory, endive, watercress, chives, shallots, parsley, tarragon, chervil, scallion tops, Chinese cabbage, radishes, hearts of palm.

Serve with Bleu Cheese Dressing*.

PICKLED CUCUMBER SALAD*
•
SALADE NIÇOISE

SERVES 4

(1 serving=2 vegetable exchanges, 1 bread exchange, 1 meat exchange, and ½ fat exchange)

Lettuce leaves
4 small tomatoes, quartered
2 cups diced cooked potatoes
2 cups cooked green beans, cut in
  strips

4 hard-cooked eggs, quartered
Tangy Salad Dressing*

On a bed of lettuce arrange mounds of tomatoes, potatoes, and green beans. Garnish with hard-cooked eggs. Serve with Tangy Salad Dressing*.

TOMATO ASPIC

SERVES 8

(1 serving=1 vegetable exchange)

2 envelopes unflavored gelatin   ½ teaspoon celery seed
¼ cup cold water   1 teaspoon salt
½ cup boiling water   1 tablespoon lemon juice
4 cups tomato juice   Salad greens
1 tablespoon grated onion

Soak gelatin in cold water. Dissolve in boiling water. Combine tomato juice, onion, celery seed, and salt. Simmer 15 minutes. Add lemon juice and gelatin. Stir until dissolved. Pour into mold and chill. Unmold on serving plate and garnish with salad greens.

TOMATO SLICES WITH BASIL

SERVES 8

(1 serving=1½ vegetable exchanges)

4 large beefsteak tomatoes
2 or 3 leaves fresh basil, minced, or ½ teaspoon dried
2 purple Italian onions, sliced

Wash the tomatoes and slice them. Sprinkle with basil. Let the tomatoes stand at least 2 hours before serving so that the basil flavor penetrates. Serve with onions.

STUFFED TOMATO SALAD

SERVES 4

(1 serving=1 meat exchange and 1 vegetable exchange)

4 small tomatoes
1 cup low-fat cottage cheese
1 tablespoon chopped chives

1 teaspoon salt
Lettuce leaves

Scoop out the center of the tomatoes. Combine cottage cheese, chives, and salt and mix. Fill the tomatoes with the cottage cheese mixture. Serve on a bed of lettuce.

FRUIT SALAD SUGGESTIONS

In making a fruit salad, there are a few rules to observe. The fruit should be ripe but not too ripe. It should be served cold. It should be kept in large enough pieces to preserve its identity. Section grapefruits, slice oranges, cut melons into balls or slices, and leave all berries whole. If the fruit is combined with cheese or meat of any kind, those ingredients should also be cold and easy to identify. In making a molded salad never boil gelatin and never add fresh pineapple to it.

A salad plate should have a light and airy touch—do not follow too definite a pattern. Here are some combinations:

½ cup sectioned grapefruit
½ cup thinly sliced onion

Serve on a bed of lettuce. (1 vegetable exchange and 1 fruit exchange)

½ cup sectioned grapefruit
⅛ an avocado, sliced

Serve on a bed of endive. (1 fruit exchange and 1 fat exchange)

½ orange, sliced
¼ cup thinly sliced, fresh
   pineapple artificially sweetened
   and mixed with fresh mint

½ cup thinly sliced honeydew
   melon
½ fresh peach, quartered

Serve on a bed of watercress and top with ¼ cup artificially sweetened lime sherbet. (2½ fruit exchanges)

1 small orange, sliced
¼ cup sectioned grapefruit

¼ cup melon balls
¼ cup low-fat cottage cheese

Serve on a bed of romaine. (1 meat exchange and 2 fruit exchanges)

¼ cup sliced cantaloupe
½ fresh peach, quartered
¼ cup whole strawberries
6 fresh green grapes

¼ cup low-fat cottage cheese
   balls, rolled in freshly chopped
   mint

Serve on a bed of curly endive. (2 fruit exchanges and 1 meat exchange)

½ cup canned artichoke hearts, cut in half
½ cup sectioned grapefruit
1 small orange, thinly sliced

Arrange in sunburst fashion on a bed of lettuce. Sprinkle with chopped chives. (1 vegetable exchange and 2 fruit exchanges)

Combine lettuce, endive, and watercress, in any amount desired, with 12 green grapes. (1 fruit exchange)

Hollow out and peel a small apple. Fill with 1 tablespoon chopped celery and 1 tablespoon raisins mixed with 1 teaspoon mayonnaise flavored with lemon juice. Serve on a bed of lettuce. (1½ fruit exchanges and 1 fat exchange)

Poppy Seed Dressing* is a nice accompaniment to all fruit salads.

CANDLE SALAD

SERVES 4

(1 serving=1½ fruit exchanges)

4 slices water-packed canned
  pineapple
Lettuce leaves

2 small bananas
2 maraschino cherries

Place pineapple slice on a lettuce leaf. Cut bananas in half cross-wise. Insert a banana half in each slice of pineapple. Top banana with half a maraschino cherry.

CRANBERRY MOLD*
●
MIXED FRUIT SALAD

SERVES 6

(1 serving=1 fruit exchange and 1 fat exchange)

2 small oranges
1 small banana, sliced
1 cup diced water-packed canned
  pineapple

⅓ cup unsweetened coconut
Lettuce leaves

Peel oranges and cut into bite-size pieces. Add banana and pineapple. Chill. Add coconut and serve on a bed of lettuce.

GRAPEFRUIT GINGER SALAD

SERVES 4

(1 serving=1 fruit exchange)

1 envelope unflavored gelatin
¾ cup water
½ teaspoon granulated sugar
  substitute (substitute for 2
  tablespoons sugar)
2 tablespoons lemon juice

1 1-pound can water-packed
  grapefruit sections with liquid
¼ cup diced celery
¼ cup diced apple
¼ teaspoon ground ginger
Salad greens

Soak gelatin in ¼ cup cold water. Add ½ cup boiling water and stir until dissolved. Add sweetener and lemon juice. Drain liquid from grapefruit sections and add enough water to make 1¼ cups. Add to gelatin mixture. Chill to unbeaten egg white consistency. Fold in grapefruit, celery, apple, and ginger. Pour into mold and chill until firm. Unmold on serving platter and garnish with salad greens.

ORANGE AND CHICKEN SALAD

SERVES 4

(1 serving=2 meat exchanges, ½ fruit exchange, and
¼ vegetable exchange)

1 cup diced cooked chicken
½ cup diced celery
2 small oranges, peeled and
  sectioned

Poppy Seed Dressing*
Lettuce leaves

Combine chicken, celery, and oranges with poppy seed dressing. Chill and serve on lettuce leaves.

SPICED PEACH SALAD

SERVES 4

(1 serving=1 fruit exchange)

1 envelope unflavored gelatin	6 whole cloves
¾ teaspoon granulated sugar substitute (substitute for 3 tablespoons sugar)	1 stick cinnamon
	¼ cup vinegar
¼ teaspoon salt	1 1-pound can water-packed peaches, sliced
1¾ cups water	Salad greens

Mix gelatin, sweetener, and salt thoroughly in a saucepan. Add water, cloves, and cinnamon. Place over low heat and simmer 10 minutes. Strain and stir in vinegar. Chill to unbeaten egg white consistency. Fold in drained peaches and pour into mold. Chill until firm. Unmold on serving platter and garnish with salad greens.

When you are making a molded fruit salad, remember that some fruits float—others sink. Apples, bananas, grapefruit, fresh peaches, fresh pears, raspberries, and halved strawberries float. Those that sink are canned apricots, canned peaches, canned pears, cherries, whole strawberries, prunes, plums, oranges, and grapes.

PINEAPPLE-COTTAGE CHEESE SALAD

SERVES 4

(1 serving=1 fruit exchange, 1 meat exchange and 1 fat exchange)

8 slices water-packed canned   1 cup low-fat cottage cheese
   pineapple   4 tablespoons unsweetened
Lettuce leaves   coconut

Place 4 pineapple slices on lettuce leaves. Spread each slice with cottage cheese. Top with remaining pineapple slice and sprinkle with coconut.

SMILE SALAD

SERVES 4

(1 serving=½ fruit exchange)

4 water-packed canned peach   8 raisins
   halves   4 peanuts
Lettuce leaves   1 maraschino cherry

Place peach half on lettuce, flat side down. Make eyes with raisins, nose with peanut, and mouth with sliver of maraschino cherry.

SPARKLING SALAD

SERVES 6

(1 serving=1 fruit exchange)

1 tablespoon unflavored gelatin
2 tablespoons cold water
½ cup boiling water
1½ cups artificially sweetened lemon-lime carbonated soda
2 tablespoons lemon juice
3½ teaspoons granulated sugar substitute (substitute for ¾ cup sugar)

1 cup water-packed canned peaches, sliced
1 cup orange sections
¼ cup sliced fresh strawberries
¼ cup grapes
½ cup diced water-packed canned pineapple
Salad greens

Soften gelatin in cold water. Add boiling water, soda, lemon juice, and sweetener and cool. Chill to unbeaten egg white consistency. Fold in fruit. Pour into mold and chill until firm. Unmold on serving plate and garnish with salad greens.

WALDORF SALAD

SERVES 3

(1 serving=2 fruit exchanges and 2 fat exchanges)

3 small apples
2 tablespoons lemon juice
6 tablespoons raisins
¼ cup chopped celery

2 tablespoons mayonnaise
2 tablespoons plain yogurt (made from skim milk)
Lettuce leaves

Chop apples and sprinkle with lemon juice. Combine with raisins, celery, mayonnaise, and yogurt. Serve on lettuce leaves.

DESSERTS

Desserts play a very important role in the eating habits of children, and diabetic children are no exception. They look forward to a sweet at the end of their meals, just as many of us do. Desserts can be prepared without the use of sugar and should not present a problem to you. The use of artificial sweeteners is acceptable. They are no more undesirable, in small amounts, than is sugar—which must be used in large quantities to achieve the same sweetening power.

The artificial sweetener that I have used for the recipes in this book has approximately 10 times the sweetening power of sugar.

BAKED APPLES

Preheat oven to 375° F.   SERVES 4

(1 serving=1 fruit exchange)

4 small apples
1 teaspoon lemon juice
1 teaspoon granulated sugar
   substitute (substitute for ¼ cup
   sugar)

4 teaspoons raisins
Cinnamon

Pare 1 inch of skin from the top of the apples and core. Brush top of apples with lemon juice. Combine sweetener and raisins and fill apples. Sprinkle with cinnamon. Bake for 45 minutes.

APPLE GRAPEFRUIT COMPOTE

SERVES 6

(1 serving=1½ fruit exchanges)

3 cups grapefruit sections
3 tablespoons plus ½ teaspoon
    granulated sugar substitute
    (substitute for 2 cups plus 2
    tablespoons sugar)

3 green apples, peeled, cored, and
    quartered
⅓ cup artificially sweetened
    cranberry juice

Sprinkle grapefruit sections with ½ teaspoon sweetener. Combine 3 tablespoons sweetener, apples, and cranberry juice in a saucepan. Cover and bring to a boil. Reduce heat and simmer 10 minutes. Uncover and boil rapidly until the apples are clear and tender, about 5 minutes. Pour over grapefruit sections. Chill overnight.

APPLE ROLLS

SERVES 4

(1 serving=1 fruit exchange and 1 bread exchange)

4 small apples
1 teaspoon lemon juice
½ teaspoon granulated sugar
    substitute (substitute for 2
    tablespoons sugar)

¼ teaspoon cinnamon
Prepared pie crust mix for 1
    8-inch pie shell

Peel and chop apples. Combine with lemon juice, sweetener, and cinnamon. Allow to stand. Prepare pie crust according to package directions. Roll very thin and cut into 4 pieces. Spoon a quarter of the apple mixture onto half of each piece. Fold over other half and pinch together to close. Bake on lightly greased baking sheet for 45 to 50 minutes at 375° F. Do not preheat oven.

APPLESAUCE

YIELDS 5 CUPS

(½ cup=1 fruit exchange)

3 pounds apples
1 small lemon, sliced
1 cup water

Core apples and combine with lemon and water. Cook over medium heat for 25 minutes. Mash through a fine sieve.

Pears may be used in place of apples to make pear sauce.

APPLE SNOW

SERVES 4

(1 serving=½ fruit exchange)

4 egg whites
Pinch salt
2 cups artificially sweetened
  applesauce
½ teaspoon lemon juice

¼ teaspoon granulated sugar
  substitute (substitute for 2
  teaspoons sugar)
⅛ teaspoon cinnamon

Beat egg whites combined with salt until they stand in stiff peaks. Combine applesauce, lemon juice, and sweetener. Stir a tablespoon of beaten egg whites into applesauce, fold in remaining egg whites, and spoon into 8 sherbet glasses. Sprinkle with cinnamon.

BAKED BANANA

Preheat oven to 400° F.   SERVES 4

(1 serving=2 fruit exchanges)

4 bananas
Rum flavoring to taste

Without peeling, split bananas in half lengthwise. Scoop out the flesh and mash, reserving the peel. Flavor with rum flavoring. Put the banana puree in a pastry bag and refill the half shells with an attractive design. Bake for 10 minutes.

BANANA PUDDING

SERVES 4

(1 serving=1 fruit exchange, ⅓ milk exchange, and ¼ bread exchange)

½ cup powdered nonfat dry milk   **2 small bananas**
2 cups warm water
2½ tablespoons arrowroot
1 teaspoon granulated sugar
substitute (substitute for ¼ cup
sugar)

Place milk, water, arrowroot, and sweetener in blender. Blend for 10 seconds, add bananas, and blend until coarsely chopped. Pour into a saucepan and cook, stirring constantly, for 5 to 7 minutes. Chill before serving.

BIRTHDAY CAKE*
•
BISCUIT TORTONI*
•
CHOCOLATE BAVARIAN CREAM

SERVES 6

(1 serving=⅔ milk exchange)

1 envelope unflavored gelatin
2 tablespoons water
¼ cup cocoa
1 cup skim milk
1½ teaspoons granulated sugar substitute (substitute for ⅓ cup sugar)

½ teaspoon vanilla
1 cup nonfat dry milk
1 cup ice water

Soften gelatin in 2 tablespoons water. Mix cocoa and skim milk and heat on top of a double boiler. Add gelatin and sweetener. Stir until gelatin is dissolved. Remove from heat and add vanilla. Let stand until mixture thickens. Combine powdered milk and ice water and beat at high speed until stiff (whipped-cream consistency). Beat gelatin mixture until smooth and fold into whipped milk. Pour into mold and chill until firm.

CHOCOLATE CUPCAKES*
●
CHOCOLATE DOUBLE-DECKERS

SERVES 4

(1 serving=1½ bread exchanges and ¼ milk exchange)

12 graham crackers
1 cup low-calorie chocolate pudding, prepared according to package
   directions
Low-calorie whipped topping, prepared according to package
   directions

Top 4 graham crackers with half the pudding, top each with another graham cracker, the remaining pudding, and then the remaining graham cracker. Top with whipped topping.

A great dessert for children from two to twenty-two.

CHOCOLATE PUDDING*
●
CRANBERRY BANANAS

SERVES 6

(1 serving=1 fruit exchange)

3 bananas, sliced
2 cups artificially sweetened cranberry sauce
Cinnamon

In 6 dessert dishes, alternate layers of bananas and cranberry sauce. Chill and serve. Sprinkle with cinnamon.

BAKED CUSTARD

Preheat oven to 350° F.   SERVES 6

(1 serving=⅓ meat exchange and ⅓ milk exchange)

2 eggs
1½ teaspoons granulated sugar
    substitute (substitute for ⅓ cup
    sugar)

¼ teaspoon salt
2 cups skim milk, scalded
½ teaspoon vanilla
Nutmeg

Beat eggs, sweetener, and salt together. Stir in milk and vanilla. Pour into 6 custard cups. Sprinkle with nutmeg. Set in a pan of hot water and bake 45 to 50 minutes or until a silver knife inserted into the custard comes out clean. Remove from oven. Cool before serving.

DATE COOKIES*
●
BROILED OR BAKED GRAPEFRUIT

SERVES 6

(1 serving=1 fruit exchange)

3 grapefruit
1½ teaspoons granulated sugar substitute (substitute for ⅓ cup sugar)
2 tablespoons rum flavoring (optional)

Cut each grapefruit in half. Cut around each section to loosen the fruit from the membrane. Sprinkle each half with ¼ teaspoon sweetener and 1 teaspoon rum flavoring. Broil 5 inches from flame until bubbly or bake at 400° F. for 20 minutes.

GRAPEFRUIT COMPOTE

SERVES 8

(1 serving=1 fruit exchange)

1¼ cups water
¾ cup unsweetened grapefruit
  juice
5 teaspoons granulated sugar
  substitute (substitute for 1 cup
  sugar)

4 cups grapefruit sections

Bring water and grapefruit juice to a boil. Stir in sweetener. Pour immediately over grapefruit sections. Chill overnight.

LEMON PARFAIT

SERVES 4

(1 serving=1 meat exchange, ½ fruit exchange, and ½ fat exchange)

4 eggs, separated
3 teaspoons granulated sugar
  substitute (substitute for ⅔ cup
  sugar)

⅓ cup lemon juice
1 teaspoon grated lemon peel
¼ teaspoon cream of tartar
1 cup fresh berries, in season

Beat egg yolks on top of double boiler until very thick. Gradually add sweetener and lemon juice. Cook, stirring constantly, until very thick and fluffy, about 2 to 3 minutes. Pour into a bowl, stir in lemon peel, and chill until cool. Beat egg whites until frothy, add cream of tartar, and continue beating until stiff. Fold egg yolk mixture into egg whites. Spoon into 4 parfait glasses, alternating with fresh berries.

LEMON PUDDING

Preheat oven to 350° F. SERVES 6

(1 serving=1¼ fat exchanges, ⅓ bread exchange, ¼ milk exchange, and ½ meat exchange)

3 eggs, separated
¼ teaspoon salt
5 teaspoons granulated sugar substitute (substitute for 1 cup sugar)

⅓ cup lemon juice
2 tablespoons butter, melted
5 tablespoons flour
1½ cups skim milk

Combine egg whites, salt, and sweetener. Beat to soft-peak stage. Combine egg yolks with remaining ingredients. Beat until smooth and fold into egg whites. Pour into a greased pan, set in a hot water bath, and bake for 1 hour. Cool in pan of water.

This is a cake-type pudding and may be served warm or cold.

MERINGUE SHELLS

Preheat oven to 250° F.   YIELDS 8 SHELLS

(need not be counted as an exchange)

4 egg whites	5 teaspoons granulated sugar
¼ teaspoon cream of tartar	substitute (substitute for 1 cup
1 teaspoon vanilla	sugar)

Beat egg whites until frothy. Add cream of tartar and vanilla and beat to soft-peak stage. Add sweetener gradually and continue beating until the egg whites are stiff but not dry. Make nestlike shells on a cookie sheet. Use ⅓ cup meringue for each shell and shape them with the back of a spoon. Bake for 1 hour.

It is easier to remove the meringue shells if the cookie sheet has been greased.

Fill the shells with:

½ cup fresh fruit topped with 2 tablespoons Lemon Sauce*=1 fruit exchange. Or:

Low-calorie vanilla pudding topped with 1 tablespoon Chocolate Sauce* (need not be counted as an exchange). Or:

Chocolate Bavarian Cream* topped with low-calorie whipped topping (need not be counted as an exchange).

Meringue shells may be stored in an airtight container in the refrigerator indefinitely.

MANDARIN ORANGE GELATIN

SERVES 4

(1 serving=½ fruit exchange)

1 package artificially sweetened orange gelatin
1 cup water-packed mandarin oranges

Make gelatin according to package directions. Divide oranges among 4 dessert dishes and pour gelatin over them. Chill until set.

ORANGE SHERBET*
●
PEACHES MELBA

SERVES 6

(1 peach=1 fruit exchange)

6 peaches
1 cup water
3 tablespoons granulated sugar
substitute (substitute for 2 cups
sugar)

1 teaspoon vanilla
Orange Sauce*

Place peaches in boiling water for a few seconds and peel. Cut in half and remove stones. Combine water, sweetener, and vanilla. Bring to a boil and simmer for 5 minutes. Poach peaches in this syrup until tender, 10 to 15 minutes. Chill before serving. Serve the peaches topped with Orange Sauce*.

SPICED PEARS

SERVES 6

(1 pear=1 fruit exchange)

⅔ cup vinegar
1 cup water
3 tablespoons granulated sugar substitute (substitute for 2 cups sugar)

1 stick cinnamon
6 pears, peeled
18 whole cloves

Combine vinegar, water, sweetener, and cinnamon. Bring to a boil. Reduce heat, add pears, cover, and simmer for ½ hour. Stick each pear with 3 cloves. Chill several hours. Remove cloves before serving.

PINEAPPLE ICE

SERVES 4

(1 serving=½ fruit exchange)

1 teaspoon unflavored gelatin
3½ teaspoons granulated sugar substitute (substitute for ¾ cup sugar)
1 cup water

¼ cup lemon juice
1 cup water-packed canned crushed pineapple, drained
1 egg white, beaten

Mix gelatin, sweetener, water, lemon juice, and pineapple. Bring to a boil. Cool. Pour into a refrigerator tray and freeze to a mush. Remove from refrigerator and beat until fluffy. Fold in egg white. Return to refrigerator tray and freeze 2 to 3 hours.

PINEAPPLE-ORANGE GELATIN

SERVES 6

(1 serving=1 fruit exchange)

1 envelope unflavored gelatin
1 cup cold water
¾ teaspoon granulated sugar substitute (substitute for 3 tablespoons sugar)
2 tablespoons frozen orange juice concentrate

Juice from unsweetened pineapple chunks plus water to make 1¼ cups
1 cup unsweetened pineapple chunks, drained
2 oranges, peeled and diced
1 banana, sliced

Combine gelatin and water in a saucepan and heat until gelatin dissolves. Add sweetener, orange juice, and liquid. Chill until it begins to thicken. Fold in fruit. Chill until set.

PINEAPPLE PUDDING

SERVES 4

(1 serving=1½ fruit exchanges)

3 cups water-packed pineapple chunks
1 teaspoon granulated sugar substitute (substitute for ¼ cup sugar)
2 tablespoons arrowroot

Place 2 cups pineapple chunks, sweetener, and arrowroot in blender. Blend for 20 seconds. Pour into saucepan and cook 5 to

7 minutes, stirring constantly. Add remaining pineapple and stir until blended. Chill before serving.

POPSICLES*
•
PUMPKIN CUSTARD* WITH WHIPPED TOPPING*
•
RASPBERRY-APRICOT SOUFFLÉ

SERVES 6

(1 serving=1 fruit exchange)

3 egg whites
2 cups fresh raspberries
¼ teaspoon granulated sugar substitute (substitute for 2 teaspoons sugar)

⅛ teaspoon ginger
⅛ teaspoon cinnamon
6 water-packed canned apricot halves

Beat egg whites until they form stiff peaks. Fold in raspberries, sweetener, ginger, and cinnamon. Spoon into 6 sherbet glasses and top with apricot halves.

RICE CUSTARD

SERVES 6

(1 serving=⅓ milk exchange, ½ fruit exchange, 1 bread exchange, and ⅓ meat exchange)

⅔ cup nonfat dry milk

1½ cups cold water

2 eggs

5 teaspoons granulated sugar substitute (substitute for 1 cup sugar)

Grated rind of ½ orange

1 teaspoon vanilla

6 tablespoons raisins

½ teaspoon nutmeg

3 cups cooked rice

Mix milk and water. Add eggs and sweetener and beat until frothy. Add remaining ingredients. Pour into casserole and bake at 350° F. for 50 minutes. Do not preheat oven.

RICE PUDDING

Preheat oven to 325° F.   SERVES 6

(1 serving=½ meat exchange, ¼ fat exchange, ½ bread exchange, ½ fruit exchange, and ⅓ milk exchange)

3 eggs, slightly beaten

2 cups skim milk

1½ cups cooked rice

2½ teaspoons granulated sugar substitute (substitute for ½ cup sugar)

6 tablespoons raisins

1 teaspoon vanilla

½ teaspoon salt

Cinnamon

Combine all ingredients except cinnamon and mix until well blended. Bake for 25 minutes. Stir and sprinkle with cinnamon. Continue baking 20 to 25 minutes or until a knife inserted in the center comes out clean.

STRAWBERRY SPONGE

SERVES 6

(1 serving=⅓ fruit exchange)

1 envelope unflavored gelatin
½ cup cold water
2½ teaspoons granulated sugar
   substitute (substitute for ½ cup
   sugar)

1½ tablespoons lemon juice
2 cups crushed strawberries
2 egg whites

Soften gelatin in cold water. Add sweetener and lemon juice. Heat over low heat until gelatin dissolves. Remove from heat and add strawberries. Let stand until mixture begins to thicken. Beat until light and fluffy. Beat egg whites until they stand in stiff peaks and fold them into gelatin mixture. Spoon into 6 sherbet glasses and chill until firm.

VANILLA PUDDING

SERVES 4

(1 serving=½ milk exchange, ½ meat exchange, ¼ fat exchange, and ¼ bread exchange)

⅔ cup nonfat dry milk
2 cups water
1 teaspoon granulated sugar
   substitute (substitute for ¼ cup
   sugar)

2½ tablespoons cornstarch
¼ teaspoon salt
2 eggs, separated
1 teaspoon vanilla

Combine dry milk with 1¾ cups water in a saucepan. Heat over low heat. Beat together sweetener, cornstarch, salt, egg yolks, and ¼ cup water. Pour into hot milk and cook over low heat, stirring constantly, until thickened. Remove from heat and add vanilla. Cool for 10 minutes. Fold in stiffly beaten egg whites.

WATERMELON BOWL*

BEVERAGES

Man does not live by bread alone, he also needs water. But we do not drink much water anymore, and to meet this need we disguise water in a variety of forms. This is especially true of children. We are all familiar with their constant requests for a cola drink, an orange drink, or a fruit punch. They are always thirsty. You should be thankful for "diet soda." If your child knows that it is a "free food," it will keep him out of a lot of trouble when he is on his own. To show you how much trouble, look at the sugar content of the more popular soft drinks:

1 teaspoon	=	5 grams
12 oz. cola drink	=	38 grams
12 oz. fruit-flavored soda	=	42 grams
12 oz. ginger ale	=	28 grams
12 oz. root beer	=	35 grams

Meanwhile, here are some beverages that you may want to have on hand at home. If you keep those that are "free foods" in a separate place, your child can drink them without having to ask for permission. One step toward independence for the two of you.

For those special occasions like football games, Halloween parties, or after skiing serve:

SPICY APPLE CIDER*
•
BANANA MILK SHAKE

SERVES 1

(1 serving=1 milk exchange and 1 fruit exchange)

1 cup skim milk
½ banana
¼ teaspoon vanilla

Put all ingredients into blender. Cover and blend for 20 seconds.

COCOA

SERVES 4

(1 cup=1 milk exchange)

4 tablespoons cocoa   **4 cups skim milk**
Pinch salt
1½ teaspoons granulated sugar
  substitute (substitute for ⅓ cup
  sugar)

Combine cocoa, salt, and sweetener in saucepan. Add ¼ cup milk and stir to form a smooth paste. Add remaining milk. Heat, stirring constantly. Do not boil. Remove from heat and beat with rotary beater until foamy. Top with low-calorie whipped topping.

Cinnamon may be used instead of salt to flavor cocoa.

No holiday gathering is complete without a glass of eggnog.

EGGNOG

SERVES 12

(½ cup=¼ milk exchange and ¼ meat exchange)

6 eggs, separated
2½ teaspoons granulated sugar substitute (substitute for ½ cup sugar)

6 cups skim milk
2 teaspoons rum flavoring, or to taste
Nutmeg

Beat egg yolks until they are thick and light in color. Add sweetener and chill. Pour into punch bowl. Slowly stir in milk and rum flavoring. Beat egg whites until stiff and fold them into mixture. Sprinkle the eggnog with nutmeg.

FRUIT PUNCH

SERVES 8

(1 cup=¾ fruit exchange)

2 tea bags
1 cup boiling water
3 tablespoons granulated sugar substitute (substitute for 2 cups sugar)
1 cup lemon juice

2 cups orange juice
1 cup artificially sweetened cranberry juice
3 cups artificially sweetened carbonated lemon-lime soda

Steep tea bags in boiling water for 5 minutes. Add sweetener. Chill. Add remaining ingredients.

HOT CHOCOLATE

SERVES 4

(1 cup=1 milk exchange)

4 cups skim milk
1 envelope low-calorie chocolate-flavored pudding

Blend ¼ cup milk with pudding. Add remaining milk and heat, stirring constantly. Store in covered container. Hot chocolate may thicken slightly when refrigerated, but it will liquefy when heated. Top with low-calorie whipped topping.

Diabetics should not consume more than 1 serving of chocolate per day.

ICED COFFEE

(need not be counted as an exchange)

Make coffee doubly strong; use 2 tablespoons instead of 1 per cup. Chill freshly brewed coffee in a china or glass pot. Pour it into glasses filled with cracked ice. Sweeten to taste with artificial sweetener.

ICED COFFEE COOLER

(need not be counted as an exchange)

Fill a glass with cracked ice ¾ full with cooled double-strength coffee. Fill to the top with club soda. Stir and serve.

SPICED ICED COFFEE

(need not be counted as an exchange)

Add 5 whole cloves, 5 whole allspice, and 1 stick cinnamon to a quart of hot double-strength coffee. Let it stand for 1 hour. Strain and pour it into glasses filled with cracked ice. Sweeten to taste, using artificial sweetener.

ICED TEA*
•
PINK LEMONADE*
•
LEMON PUNCH

SERVES 5

(1 cup=1 fruit exchange)

2 tea bags
1 cup boiling water
2½ tablespoons granulated sugar
   substitute (substitute for 1½
   cups sugar)

1 cup lemon juice
1 cup unsweetened pineapple juice
2 cups artificially sweetened
   carbonated lemon-lime soda

Steep tea bags in boiling water for 5 minutes. Add sweetener. Chill. Add remaining ingredients.

LIME MIST

SERVES 4

(need not be counted as an exchange)

½ cup lime juice
1 teaspoon granulated sugar substitute (substitute for ¼ cup sugar)

2 cups water
2 cups artificially sweetened carbonated lime soda

Combine lime juice, sweetener, and water. Chill. Before serving add lime soda.

If your child is not feeling well or if he is pressed for time, he may enjoy drinking his breakfast:

NUTRITION SNACK

SERVES 2

(1 serving=½ milk exchange, 1½ fruit exchanges, ¼ fat exchange, and ½ meat exchange)

1 cup skim milk
½ cup orange juice
1 banana
1 egg

¼ teaspoon vanilla
¼ teaspoon granulated sugar substitute (substitute for 1 tablespoon sugar) (optional)

Combine all ingredients in blender and blend for 20 seconds.

ORANGEADE

SERVES 4

(1 cup=2 fruit exchanges)

3 cups orange juice   1 orange, sliced
1 cup lemon juice
3 teaspoons granulated sugar
   substitute (substitute for ⅔ cup
   sugar)

Combine all ingredients and chill.

ORANGE FROST

SERVES 2

(1 serving=1 fruit exchange, ½ meat exchange, and ¼ fat exchange)

1 cup orange juice   6 ice cubes
1 egg
¼ teaspoon granulated sugar
   substitute (substitute for 1
   tablespoon sugar)

Combine all ingredients in blender and blend for 20 seconds.

ORANGE MILK SHAKE

SERVES 2

(1 serving=½ milk exchange, ½ fruit exchange, ½ meat exchange, and ¼ fat exchange)

1 cup skim milk
½ cup orange juice
1 egg
¼ teaspoon vanilla

¼ teaspoon granulated sugar substitute (substitute for 1 tablespoon sugar) (optional)

Combine all ingredients in blender and blend for 20 seconds.

PARTY PUNCH*
●
SPICED TEA

SERVES 4

(need not be counted as an exchange)

3 cups boiling water
3 tea bags
½ teaspoon whole cloves
1 stick cinnamon

1½ teaspoons granulated sugar substitute (substitute for ⅓ cup sugar)
½ cup orange juice

Combine boiling water, tea bags, spices, and sweetener. Steep for 5 minutes. Strain. Add orange juice and heat but do not boil. Serve hot.

VEGETABLE COCKTAIL

SERVES 2

(1 serving=2 vegetable exchanges)

1 cup tomato juice
1 rib celery, diced
1 carrot, diced
½ small onion, diced

1 tablespoon lemon juice
½ teaspoon salt
Dash pepper
Dash Worcestershire sauce

Combine all ingredients in blender and blend 20 seconds.

SNACKS

As your child matures you are not going to be able to stand over him and select his diet. He will soon be out with the crowd eager to try his wings. The knowledge that you impart to him in his youth will stand him in good stead in the years ahead. Habits formed in childhood do carry over into adult life. So start to allow him to make some choices in his daily diet. Snacks are a good place to allow for "free choice." A special storage place for these foods that are acceptable is a good way to begin. Later you may want to involve your child in the actual preparation of foods that are suitable for between-meal snacks.

Plan to divide his day into three meals and two snacks. One snack after school and one before bed is a pretty good rule. This way you can calculate what he has consumed throughout the day and allow for snack times to balance the allotted exchanges. There is an exchange scoreboard (Appendix H) that you can use to simplify this task, one that will also involve your child in the daily computation. It will help him to abide by his own rules and give him some flexibility in choosing certain foods.

APPLE CHIPS

Preheat oven to 325° F.

(½ cup=1 fruit exchange)

Coarsely shred apples and put them on a lightly greased baking sheet. Bake for 20 minutes or until dry. Remove with pancake turner and store in an airtight container.

BANANA TOAST

SERVES 4

(1 serving=1 bread exchange and 1 fruit exchange)

4 slices bread
2 small bananas

Toast bread and mash ½ banana on each slice of toast. Place under broiler to brown.

STUFFED CELERY

(1 12- to 15-inch rib celery=1 vegetable exchange)

Mixtures for stuffing celery may be made with:

Low-fat cream cheese moistened with a little skim milk. Chopped chives or raisins may be added for variety.
(1 tablespoon cream cheese=1 fat exchange)
(1 tablespoon raisins=½ fruit exchange)

Low-fat Roquefort or bleu cheese mashed with a little skim milk and mixed with chopped chives.
(2 tablespoons=1 meat exchange)

Peanut butter.
(2 tablespoons=1 meat exchange and 2½ fat exchanges)

ROASTED CHESTNUTS

Preheat oven to 400° F.

(6 chestnuts=1 fat exchange)

Make a small cut on the side of each chestnut. Place chestnuts in a single layer on a baking sheet. Roast for 30 minutes. Shake occasionally.

DATE COOKIES

Preheat oven to 350° F.   YIELDS 36 COOKIES

(1 cookie=¼ fruit exchange and ⅔ fat exchange)

8 tablespoons raisins
12 dates, chopped
1 cup water
½ cup butter
2 eggs
2½ teaspoons granulated sugar
   substitute (substitute for ½ cup
   sugar)

1 teaspoon vanilla
1 cup flour
1 teaspoon baking soda
¼ teaspoon cinnamon

Combine raisins, dates, and water and boil for 3 minutes, stirring constantly. Cool. Cream butter and add eggs, sweetener, and vanilla. Blend until light and creamy. Sift flour, baking soda, and cinnamon. Add dry ingredients alternately with date mixture, to the butter mixture. Chill several hours. Drop from teaspoon onto greased baking pan. Bake for 10 minutes.

DEVILED EGGS

SERVES 12

(1 serving=½ meat exchange and ¼ fat exchange)

6 eggs
1 teaspoon prepared mustard

1 tablespoon mayonnaise
Salt and pepper to taste

Simmer (do not boil) eggs for 15 to 20 minutes. Cool eggs by plunging them, at once, into cold water. Remove shells and split eggs in half lengthwise. Remove the yolks. Mash yolks with mustard and mayonnaise. Season to taste. Stuff the whites.

For variety:

Garnish with paprika. Or:
Add 1 tablespoon chopped unsweetened pickle. Or:
Mash 6 egg yolks with 2 tablespoons cream cheese moistened with milk and add a bit of anchovy paste. (Cream cheese need not be counted as an exchange.) Or:
Season with curry powder.

FRESH FRUITS

Fresh fruits in season are an ideal snack food. They are rich in minerals and vitamins. They are always a delight to eat because of the variety of their textures and flavors. The following fruits may be used for 1 fruit exchange.

1 small apple	12 grapes
2 medium apricots	½ small mango
½ small banana	Melons:
Berries:	¼ small cantaloupe
½ cup blackberries	⅛ medium honeydew melon
½ cup blueberries	1 cup watermelon
½ cup raspberries	1 small orange
¾ cup strawberries	1 medium peach
10 large cherries	1 medium pear
1 fresh fig	2 medium plums
½ grapefruit	1 medium tangerine

GELATIN

SERVES 4

(need not be counted as an exchange)

2 cups water
1 envelope low-calorie artificially sweetened gelatin

Boil 1 cup water and add to gelatin. Stir until dissolved. Add 1 cup cold water. Chill until set.

For variety:

Chill until slightly thickened. Add 1 cup plain yogurt (made from skim milk). Beat until light and fluffy. Chill. Makes 8 servings.

(need not be counted as an exchange)

Chill until thickened. Fold in 1 small orange, sectioned, or ½ small banana, sliced. Makes 5 servings.

(need not be counted as an exchange)

MARBLES

YIELDS 24 MARBLES

(1 marble=1 fruit exchange)

12 dried figs, finely chopped   **Unsweetened shredded coconut**
16 dried prunes, finely chopped   **(optional)**
8 tablespoons raisins

Combine figs, prunes, and raisins and roll into 24 balls. Roll in shredded coconut or leave plain, as desired. (1 tablespoon coconut=1 fat exchange)

PEANUT BUTTER BALLS

YIELDS 32 BALLS

(1 ball=1 fat exchange and ¼ meat exchange)

1 cup peanut butter
3½ ounces nonfat dry milk
2½ teaspoons granulated sugar
    substitute (substitute for ½
    cup sugar)

1 teaspoon sesame seeds (optional)
5 tablespoons water
1 cup unsweetened shredded
    coconut

Combine all ingredients except coconut. Form into 32 balls. Dip balls into warm water and roll in coconut.

MINIATURE PIZZAS

SERVES 8

(1 serving=¼ vegetable exchange, ½ meat exchange, ¼ fat exchange, and 1 bread exchange)

4 English muffins, split
1 cup Tomato Sauce*
Oregano

Basil
Salt and pepper to taste
½ cup grated mozzarella cheese

Toast muffins. Top each half with 2 tablespoons tomato sauce seasoned with oregano, basil, salt, and pepper. Sprinkle each with 1 tablespoon cheese. Broil until brown and bubbly.

POPCORN*

•

CHEESE POPCORN

(½ cup need not be counted as an exchange)

To 1 recipe hot popcorn* add 3 tablespoons grated Parmesan cheese.

RAISIN-NUT POPCORN

(½ cup=½ fruit exchange and ½ fat exchange)

Combine 1 cup of popcorn with 2 tablespoons raisins and 10 whole peanuts.

APPLE POPSICLES

YIELDS 12 POPSICLES

(1 Popsicle=⅔ fruit exchange)

2 cups apple juice
1 envelope unflavored gelatin
1 cup unsweetened applesauce

¾ teaspoon granulated sugar substitute (substitute for 3 tablespoons sugar)

Pour 1 cup boiling apple juice over gelatin. Stir until dissolved. Add 1 cup cold apple juice, applesauce, and sweetener. Stir to blend well. Pour into Popsicle molds and freeze.

If you do not have Popsicle molds you can use a paper cup and insert a stick when the mixture is partially frozen. I use plastic molds called "Ice Tups" that are available from Tupperware. When it is frozen the Popsicle may be a little hard to get out of the mold, so just briefly run the mold under some cold water.

BANANA POPSICLES

YIELDS 6 POPSICLES

(1 Popsicle=¼ milk exchange and ⅓ fruit exchange)

1 small banana
1½ cups skim milk
Dash nutmeg

Combine all ingredients in blender and blend for 20 seconds. Pour into Popsicle molds and freeze.

FRUIT-FLAVORED POPSICLES

YIELDS 16 POPSICLES

(need not be counted as an exchange)

1 package cherry-flavored
  artificially sweetened gelatin
4 cups water
1 package cherry-flavored
  unsweetened soft drink mix

5 teaspoons granulated sugar
substitute (substitute for 1 cup
sugar)

Dissolve gelatin in 1 cup boiling water. Add remaining ingredients. Stir until dissolved. Pour into Popsicle molds and freeze.

Any other fruit flavors may be used. Red and orange seem to be children's favorites.

FUDGESICLES

YIELDS 8 POPSICLES

(1 Popsicle=¼ milk exchange)

2 ounces low-calorie artificially sweetened chocolate pudding
2 cups skim milk

Gradually add milk to pudding mix. Stir over medium heat until mixture comes to a boil. Pour into Popsicle molds and freeze.

FROSTY ORANGE POPSICLES

YIELDS 6 POPSICLES

(1 Popsicle=⅓ fruit exchange)

1 cup orange juice
1 egg
¼ teaspoon granulated sugar substitute (substitute for 1 tablespoon sugar)

Combine all ingredients in blender and blend for 20 seconds. Pour into Popsicle molds and freeze.

CREAMY ORANGE POPSICLES

YIELDS 8 POPSICLES

(1 Popsicle need not be counted as an exchange)

1 cup skim milk
½ cup orange juice
1 egg
¼ teaspoon vanilla

¼ teaspoon granulated sugar substitute (substitute for 1 tablespoon sugar)

Combine all ingredients in blender and blend for 20 seconds. Pour into Popsicle molds and freeze.

GRAHAM CRACKERS

(1 cracker=½ bread exchange)

Most children enjoy graham crackers served plain with a glass of milk. For variety:

Spread with 1 tablespoon low-fat cream cheese (add 1 fat exchange). Or:

Spread with 1 tablespoon peanut butter (add ½ meat exchange and 1¼ fat exchanges). Or:

Frost with Chocolate Coating.*

RAW VEGETABLES

(½ cup=1 vegetable exchange)

Raw vegetables can be stored in the refrigerator and make an ideal snack that will provide minerals and vitamins so necessary for growing children.

CONDIMENTS, DRESSINGS, AND SAUCES

This chapter is a collection of those usually prepared foods that are not acceptable for your diabetic child's consumption and therefore must be prepared "from scratch." Most already prepared sauces, salad dressings, and condiments contain a great deal of sugar or fat. Since the amounts are not listed, it is impossible for you to calculate the fat exchanges or to know how much sugar they contain. It is better to be on the safe side and to prepare your own. The recipes are simple, take little time to prepare, and are well worth the effort.

CATSUP

YIELDS 2 PINTS

(1 tablespoon need not be counted as an exchange)

25 medium tomatoes
1 medium onion, chopped
¼ teaspoon cayenne
5 teaspoons granulated sugar
   substitute (substitute for 1 cup
   sugar)

1 cup white vinegar
1½ teaspoons whole cloves
1 stick cinnamon
1 teaspoon celery seed
4 teaspoons salt

Core and quarter tomatoes and place in a large pan with onion and cayenne. Bring to a boil and cook for 15 minutes, stirring occasionally. Strain tomatoes through a coarse sieve. Add sweetener and simmer for 2 hours.

Combine vinegar, cloves, cinnamon, and celery seed. Cover and bring to a boil. Remove from heat and let stand. When tomato juice has finished simmering, strain vinegar into the tomato juice and add salt. Simmer 30 minutes longer. Stir frequently.

CHILI SAUCE

YIELDS 1 QUART

(1 tablespoon need not be counted as an exchange)

18 medium tomatoes
1 bunch celery, finely chopped
1¼ cups finely chopped onion
1¼ cups finely chopped green
    pepper
3 sticks cinnamon
¾ teaspoon ground cloves

1½ teaspoons dry mustard
4 tablespoons granulated brown
    sugar substitute (substitute for
    2¼ cups brown sugar)
2 cups cider vinegar
2 tablespoons salt

Peel, core, and quarter tomatoes. Cook for 15 minutes. Drain off half the juice (reserve for drinking or cooking). Add celery, onion, and green pepper. Simmer 1½ hours. Add remaining ingredients and cook 1½ hours. Remove cinnamon.

CHOCOLATE COATING*
●
CHOCOLATE FROSTING*
●
COATING FOR CHICKEN*
●
COCKTAIL SAUCE

(2 tablespoons need not be counted as an exchange)

1 cup Tomato Sauce*
½ cup Chili Sauce*
1 tablespoon lemon juice
1 tablespoon horseradish

¼ teaspoon salt
Dash pepper
Few drops Tabasco

Combine all ingredients and mix well.

BLEU CHEESE DRESSING

(4 tablespoons need not be counted as an exchange)

½ teaspoon granulated sugar
   substitute (substitute for 2
   tablespoons sugar)
1 cup beef bouillon

2 tablespoons Chili Sauce*
2 tablespoons vinegar
1 tablespoon grated onion
1 ounce bleu cheese, crumbled

Combine all ingredients and mix until blended.

FRENCH DRESSING

(need not be counted as an exchange)

⅓ cup water
1½ teaspoons cornstarch
⅓ cup tomato juice
⅓ cup vinegar
¼ teaspoon granulated sugar
  substitute (substitute for 1
  tablespoon sugar)

½ teaspoon salt
½ teaspoon dry mustard
1 small clove garlic, crushed
Dash Tabasco

Combine water and cornstarch and stir until smooth. Add remaining ingredients and boil for 1 minute. Cool to room temperature. Refrigerate until ready to use.

Try this dressing on any vegetable salad.

POPPY SEED DRESSING

(need not be counted as an exchange)

1 teaspoon unflavored gelatin
1 tablespoon cold water
¼ cup boiling water
2½ teaspoons granulated sugar
  substitute (substitute for ½ cup
  sugar)
½ teaspoon salt

½ cup lemon juice
⅛ teaspoon dry mustard
⅛ teaspoon pepper
½ clove garlic, crushed
1 teaspoon chopped chives
¼ teaspoon poppy seeds

Soften gelatin in cold water. Dissolve in boiling water. Add sweetener and salt. Cool. Combine remaining ingredients and add to gelatin mixture. Blend thoroughly and refrigerate. Remove from refrigerator 1 hour before serving. The flavor is best at room temperature.

Serve with fruit salads.

TANGY SALAD DRESSING

(4 tablespoons need not be counted as an exchange)

½ teaspoon granulated sugar substitute (substitute for 2 tablespoons sugar)
1 cup tomato juice
2 tablespoons lemon juice

½ small onion, grated
½ teaspoon garlic powder
2 teaspoons prepared horseradish
Dash Tabasco sauce

Combine all ingredients and mix until well blended.

YOGURT SALAD DRESSING

(4 tablespoons need not be counted as an exchange)

2 tablespoons lemon juice
⅔ cup plain yogurt (made from skim milk)

Salt and pepper to taste
1 tablespoon finely chopped parsley

Blend together lemon juice and yogurt. Season to taste. Sprinkle with parsley.

DEVILED EGGS*
●
PICKLED EGGS

(1 egg=1 meat exchange and ½ fat exchange)

Simmer eggs for 15 to 20 minutes. Cool eggs by plunging them at once into cold water. Peel eggs and cover them with a mixture of equal parts of beet juice and vinegar. A sliced onion and a few whole cloves may be added. Marinate in the refrigerator for 2 days.

ORANGE GLAZE*
●
MOCK HOLLANDAISE*
●
FRENCH MUSTARD

(need not be counted as an exchange)

1 onion, sliced
1 cup vinegar
1 teaspoon salt
1 teaspoon pepper

¼ teaspoon granulated sugar substitute (substitute for 1 tablespoon sugar)
½ cup dry mustard

Soak onion in vinegar overnight. Discard onion and pour vinegar into a saucepan. Mix together salt, pepper, sweetener, and mustard. Add enough vinegar to form a smooth paste. Heat remaining vinegar and slowly add mustard mixture, stirring until smooth. Bring to a boil and cook for 5 minutes. Remove from heat and let stand overnight. Store in a covered jar.

BARBECUE SAUCE*

●

CHOCOLATE SAUCE

(2 tablespoons need not be counted as an exchange)

1 tablespoon butter
2 tablespoons cocoa
1 tablespoon cornstarch
Dash salt
1 cup skim milk

1½ teaspoons granulated sugar
 substitute (substitute for ⅓ cup
 sugar)
½ teaspoon vanilla

Melt butter. Combine cocoa, cornstarch, and salt and add to melted butter. Stir until smooth. Add milk and sweetener and cook, stirring constantly, until slightly thickened. Remove from heat and add vanilla. Set in a pan of ice water and stir until sauce is cold and thick, about 5 minutes.

LEMON SAUCE

(2 tablespoons need not be counted as an exchange)

3 tablespoons cornstarch
3½ teaspoons granulated sugar
 substitute (substitute for ¾ cup
 sugar)
¼ teaspoon salt

⅛ teaspoon nutmeg
6 tablespoons lemon juice
1 tablespoon butter
1½ cups boiling water
2 teaspoons grated lemon peel

Combine cornstarch, sweetener, salt, and nutmeg in saucepan. Add lemon juice and stir until smooth. Add butter and boiling water and cook, stirring constantly, until thickened. Add lemon peel. Serve warm.

MINT SAUCE*

•

ORANGE SAUCE

(2 tablespoons need not be counted as an exchange)

3 tablespoons cornstarch
¼ teaspoon salt
1½ teaspoons granulated sugar
  substitute (substitute for ⅓ cup
  sugar)

1 cup orange juice
1 cup boiling water
2 tablespoons grated orange peel

Combine cornstarch, salt, and sweetener in a saucepan. Add orange juice and stir until smooth. Add boiling water and bring to a boil, stirring constantly. Boil 2 minutes. Add orange peel. Serve warm.

STRAWBERRY SAUCE

(3 tablespoons strawberries=¼ fruit exchange)

2 cups strawberries
1¼ teaspoons granulated sugar substitute (substitute for 4 tablespoons
  sugar)

Place strawberries and sweetener in blender and blend 20 seconds.

TOMATO SAUCE

YIELDS 5 CUPS

(½ cup=1 vegetable exchange)

4 medium onions, chopped
2 cloves garlic, minced
2 tablespoons olive oil
4 pounds tomatoes, sliced

2 6-ounce cans tomato paste
1 teaspoon dried basil
1 teaspoon salt
Dash pepper

Sauté onion and garlic in oil until onions are transparent. Stir in remaining ingredients. Cook over a low flame, stirring frequently, for 1 hour. Strain through a fine sieve.

WHIPPED TOPPING

(need not be counted as an exchange)

½ cup ice water
½ cup nonfat dry milk
3 tablespoons lemon juice

¾ teaspoon granulated sugar
substitute (substitute for 3
tablespoons sugar)

Chill bowl and beaters. Combine ice water and dry milk and beat at high speed until it stands in peaks, about 5 minutes. Add lemon juice and sweetener. Chill 1 hour.

FESTIVE OCCASIONS

There were real fireworks in our house when I announced that we were not going to have our traditional Fourth of July picnic. I really didn't know how to put it all together. Sherry had officially been pronounced diabetic on June 15. The exchanges were still a maze of confusion to me, and I knew that Sherry would eat everything in sight. She had already been through a few bouts with insulin shock, and, to say the least, I was a bit unnerved. My children are anything but traditional, except for holidays. Then, they are like old grandmothers—nothing can ever change. My son even checks the dining room table at Christmas to make certain that I have not forgotten an accustomed eating utensil or decoration. I really was not concerned about Thanksgiving and Christmas. I had four and five months to test recipes for those occasions. But, the Fourth of July was a different matter! My son threatened to leave home and I didn't think that was too bad an idea. One less persuader would have helped to ease my conscience a bit. Unfortunately, he didn't go, he just invited Grandma to join in our festivities. Sherry played the martyr. She would not come out of her room, except to eat. You'd think that I personally invented diabetes. On the contrary, nobody in my family ever had the disease and I did not feel the least bit guilty about being the cause.

Well, guess who won? I felt as if I should have been selected for the Mother of the Year award as we gathered our wares, on a gorgeous, sunny Fourth of July, and set off on our annual celebration. Our picnic basket consisted of:

Barbecued Chicken
Cherry Tomatoes   Celery Curls
Pickled Cucumber Salad
Baked Beans
Chocolate Pudding   Hand Fruit
Iced Tea

BARBECUED CHICKEN

Preheat oven to 325° F.   SERVES 6

(1 ounce chicken=1 meat exchange)

Place 6 chicken breasts or 6 legs in a baking dish. Cover with barbecue sauce (below). Cover and bake for 45 minutes. Remove cover and bake another 15 minutes at 400°.

BARBECUE SAUCE

(need not be counted as an exchange)

1 cup bouillon	½ clove garlic, minced
1 tablespoon cornstarch	¼ cup minced onion
¼ cup vinegar	¼ teaspoon Tabasco sauce
½ teaspoon prepared mustard	1 bay leaf
½ teaspoon Worcestershire sauce	¼ teaspoon whole cloves
2 tablespoons Chili Sauce*	½ teaspoon granulated sugar
1 tablespoon lemon juice	substitute (substitute for 2
Grated rind of ½ lemon	tablespoons sugar)

Mix bouillon and cornstarch and cook over low heat until smooth and thickened. Add remaining ingredients and cook until onion is soft.

CELERY CURLS

(½ cup=1 vegetable exchange)

Break a stalk of celery into ribs. Cut each rib in 3-inch lengths. At the end of each piece make 4 lengthwise cuts to the center. Crisp in ice water.

PICKLED CUCUMBER SALAD

SERVES 6

(½ cup=1 vegetable exchange)

2 large cucumbers (8-inch) or 3
  medium (6-inch)
1 tablespoon salt
¾ cup white vinegar
¼ teaspoon granulated sugar
  substitute (substitute for 1
  tablespoon sugar)

1 teaspoon salt
¼ teaspoon pepper
2 tablespoons chopped fresh dill

Scrub the wax coating, if any, off the cucumbers and dry. Score the cucumbers lengthwise with a fork and cut them in the thinnest possible slices. The slices should be almost translucent. Arrange them in a thin layer in a shallow glass dish and sprinkle with salt. Place 2 to 3 plates on top of the cucumbers to press out the excess water and bitterness and let stand at room temperature for a couple of hours. Remove the plates, drain the cucumbers of all the liquid, dry them with paper towels, and return them to their dish. In a small bowl, beat together vinegar, sweetener, salt, and pepper. Pour over the cucumbers and sprinkle them with chopped dill. Chill for 2 or 3 hours. Just before serving drain off all of the liquid.

CHOCOLATE PUDDING

SERVES 8

(1 serving=½ milk exchange)

2 ounces low-calorie artificially sweetened chocolate pudding
4 cups skim milk

Empty pudding into saucepan. Gradually add milk. Stir over medium heat until mixture comes to a boil. Pudding thickens as it cools.

ICED TEA

SERVES 6

(need not be counted as an exchange)

6 teaspoons loose tea or 6 tea bags   **Granulated sugar substitute to**
6 cups boiling water   **taste**
1 tray ice cubes   **6 lemon wedges**

Tea should be brewed in an earthenware or china pot. Always use freshly boiled water. Allow the tea to steep for 5 minutes.

Pour tea over ice cubes. Sweeten to taste. Serve with lemon wedges.

The other contents of the picnic basket do not need recipes, but their exchange values are as follows:

Cherry Tomatoes	½ cup=1 vegetable exchange
Baked Beans, no pork (canned)	¼ cup=1 bread exchange
Hand Fruit†	1 small=1 fruit exchange
Skim Milk	1 cup=1 milk exchange

Your child has a prescribed daily allowance of food exchanges for breakfast, lunch, and dinner. On festive occasions you may have to rearrange the distribution of the exchanges to keep things in balance. Subtract the exchanges allotted for the special meal from the day's total and divide the remaining prescribed exchanges between the other two meals.

By Thanksgiving the exchanges and I were old friends and from then on it was smooth sailing right through the holidays. Meals adhered to both traditional and diabetic standards.

THANKSGIVING DINNER

Hot Tangy Bouillon

Roast Turkey   Celery Onion Stuffing

Glazed Onions   Savory Spinach

Hearts of Celery   Carrot Curls

Olives

Hot Rolls   Butter

Pumpkin Custard   Whipped Topping

† See Appendix B, Fruit Exchanges.

HOT TANGY BOUILLON

SERVES 6

(need not be counted as an exchange)

1 quart beef bouillon   1 tablespoon Worcestershire sauce
3 tablespoons lemon juice   Lemon slices

Combine first three ingredients. Heat and serve. Garnish with lemon slices.

ROAST TURKEY

Preheat oven to 325° F.   ½ POUND=1 SERVING

(1 ounce turkey=1 meat exchange)

Stuff turkey just before roasting. If stuffing is prepared the day before, refrigerate it until ready to use. Place the turkey, breast side up, on a rack in an uncovered roasting pan. Do not add water. Roast according to the following table:

Pounds	Hours
4 to 6	3 to 4
6 to 12	4 to 5
12 to 16	5 to 6
16 to 20	6 to 7½
20 to 24	7½ to 9

Plan to have the turkey finished about ½ hour before you are ready to eat. It will retain its heat if allowed to stand at room temperature and it will be easier to carve.

CELERY ONION STUFFING

SERVES 10

(½ cup=1 bread exchange and ⅓ vegetable exchange)

8 cups stale bread crumbs
1 cup minced onion
¾ cup bouillon
½ cup chopped celery
½ tablespoon sage
½ cup chopped celery leaves

½ tablespoon thyme
½ teaspoon crumbled bay leaf
½ clove garlic, finely chopped
1 tablespoon salt
½ teaspoon pepper

Heat the bread crumbs in a slow oven until they are dried but not browned. Add onion to bouillon and cook until tender. Add crumbs and remaining ingredients and cook 2 to 3 minutes, stirring constantly. Cool the stuffing before filling turkey. Fill loosely to allow for expansion during cooking.

GLAZED ONIONS

SERVES 6

(½ cup=1 vegetable exchange and 1 fat exchange)

3 cups small white onions, peeled
2 tablespoons butter
⅔ cup chicken bouillon

¼ teaspoon granulated sugar substitute (substitute for 1 tablespoon sugar)

Combine all ingredients. Bring to a boil, reduce heat, and simmer very slowly. Turn onions occasionally and cook until the onions are tender and the liquid is reduced to a syrupy glaze.

SAVORY SPINACH

SERVES 6

(1 serving=1 vegetable exchange and 1 fat exchange)

3 cups frozen cooked chopped
    spinach
1 tablespoon lemon juice
2 tablespoons butter

½ teaspoon salt
Dash pepper
Dash nutmeg

Combine all ingredients and heat 1 to 2 minutes.

CARROT CURLS*
•
PUMPKIN CUSTARD

Preheat oven to 350° F.   SERVES 6

(1 serving=⅓ bread exchange and ⅓ meat exchange)

2 eggs
2½ teaspoons granulated sugar
    substitute (substitute for ½ cup
    sugar)

1 cup skim milk
1 teaspoon cinnamon
1 teaspoon ground ginger
2 cups cooked pumpkin

Beat eggs and add sweetener. Add milk and spices. Combine with pumpkin. Pour into 8-inch pie plate. Bake 50 to 60 minutes or until a silver knife, inserted into center of custard, comes out clean. Remove from oven. Cool before serving. Serve with Whipped Topping.*

Also included in the dinner are the following foods that have an exchange value of:

hearts of celery: ½ cup=1 vegetable exchange;

carrot curls: ½ cup=1 vegetable exchange;

olives: 5=1 fat exchange;

rolls: 1=1 bread exchange;

butter: 1 teaspoon=1 fat exchange.

CHRISTMAS DINNER

French Onion Soup
Baked Ham with Orange Glaze
Brussels Sprouts with Pimento
Winter Squash
Cranberry Mold
Hot Rolls   Butter
Biscuit Tortoni

FRENCH ONION SOUP

SERVES 6

(1 serving=1 vegetable exchange and ½ fat exchange)

3 cups sliced onions	½ teaspoon Worcestershire sauce
3 teaspoons butter	Salt and pepper to taste
3 10½-ounce cans beef bouillon	Grated Parmesan cheese

Brown onions in butter. Add bouillon, Worcestershire, salt, and pepper and heat. Serve with a sprinkling of grated Parmesan cheese.

BAKED HAM

Preheat oven to 300° F.   ¼ POUND=1 SERVING

(1 ounce=1 meat exchange)

Place ham on a rack in a shallow pan. Select the length of time suggested for the kind and weight of the ham that you are cooking. Do not score or remove the outer rind. Do not season or baste. About ½ hour before ham is done, remove from the oven. Cut away the outer rind, leaving an even layer of fat about ¼ inch thick. Score surface in diamond design. Stud with whole cloves if desired. Spoon orange glaze (below) over the entire surface. Return to oven and finish baking.

Tenderized ham should bake 4 hours. Ready-to-eat hams should take 2 hours. Fully cooked or canned hams should be heated thoroughly. Both the flavor and the texture are improved if baked 2 hours.

Home-cured hams need soaking in cold water overnight. Then place in a kettle of cold water so the ham is just covered. Simmer 25 minutes per pound. Cool in water in which it was cooked. Then bake for 2 hours.

ORANGE GLAZE

(need not be counted as an exchange)

3½ tablespoons grated orange peel
½ cup orange juice
2 teaspoons dry mustard
2 tablespoons prepared mustard
5 teaspoons granulated sugar substitute (substitute for 1 cup sugar)

Combine all ingredients. Boil rapidly for 5 minutes. Cool to room temperature.

BRUSSELS SPROUTS WITH PIMIENTO

SERVES 6

(1 serving=1 vegetable exchange and ½ fat exchange)

3 cups brussels sprouts
1 tablespoon butter
2 ounces pimiento, diced

Clean and trim brussels sprouts. Steam over boiling water or cook them in boiling salted water until tender. Drain. Add butter and pimiento and cook 3 minutes longer.

WINTER SQUASH

SERVES 6

(1 serving=1 bread exchange and ½ fat exchange)

3 cups ½-inch slices squash
1 tablespoon butter
2 tablespoons instant minced
  onion

¾ teaspoon grated lemon peel
2 tablespoons lemon juice
¼ cup chopped fresh parsley

Steam squash over boiling water or cook in a small amount of boiling salted water until just tender. Drain. Combine butter, onion, lemon peel, and lemon juice. Heat until butter is melted. Pour over squash. Add parsley and mix thoroughly.

CRANBERRY MOLD

SERVES 6

(1 serving=1 fruit exchange and ⅓ vegetable exchange)

1 tablespoon plain gelatin
1 cup unsweetened pineapple juice
1 package cherry-flavored artificially sweetened gelatin
1 cup hot water
3½ teaspoons granulated sugar substitute (substitute for ¾ cup sugar)

1 tablespoon lemon juice
1 cup water-packed canned crushed pineapple
1 cup ground raw cranberries
1 orange and rind, finely ground
1 cup chopped celery
Salad greens

Dissolve plain gelatin in pineapple juice. Melt over hot water. Dissolve cherry gelatin in hot water. Add sweetener, lemon juice, and pineapple. Combine with plain gelatin mixture. Stir until blended. Chill to unbeaten egg white consistency. Add remaining ingredients and pour into mold. Chill until firm. Unmold on serving platter and garnish with salad greens.

BISCUIT TORTONI

SERVES 8

(1 serving=⅓ milk exchange)

1½ tablespoons lemon juice
1½ cups water
1 cup nonfat dry milk
¾ teaspoon granulated sugar substitute (substitute for 2⅔ tablespoons sugar)

½ teaspoon vanilla
½ teaspoon almond extract

Combine lemon juice and water in mixing bowl. Add dry milk and beat until stiff (whipped-cream consistency). Add sweetener, vanilla, and almond extract. Beat until well blended. Pour into refrigerator tray and freeze with refrigerator at coldest point.

Also included in the dinner are the following foods that have an exchange value of: rolls: 1=1 bread exchange; butter: 1 teaspoon=1 fat exchange.

BIRTHDAY PARTIES

With fear and trepidation I started to plan Sherry's first diabetic birthday party. Children can be cruel if their expectations are not met and I wanted this to be a happy event. Birthday celebrations in our house had always been very festive occasions. Ponies, clowns, or magicians had set the scene in the past. The party always culminated with the proper refreshments: ice cream, chocolate cake, candy, and soda. Sherry's greatest area of concern, as she counted the days until her birthday, was her inability to consume what she then considered to be her favorite foods. She simply could not understand why she was not allowed to eat ice cream, or cake, or cookies, or candy. She felt that she was being punished. Besides, who ever heard of a birthday party without a birthday cake and ice cream?

I knew that I had to divert her attention away from the traditional party fare. As a home economist for a public utility, I had taught cooking classes for young children who had not progressed far enough in their schooling to have home economics as a part of their curriculum. I realized how much they enjoyed playing chef in the kitchen and how infrequently mothers have the time or the patience to allow them to take over. So I decided to have a Chef's Birthday Party and to allow the guests to prepare the Birthday Feast. The invitations that were sent read:

Sherry is having a party.
March 17th is the day.
You are invited to help,
In a most unusual way.
So wear old clothes,
And arrive at four.
You must be on time,
If you want to know more.

Seven children were invited to this affair and I hoped that my kitchen, and I, would survive. But Sherry was excited and together we planned the menu:

Sloppy Joes

Carrot Curls   Unsweetened Pickle Slices

Birthday Cake   Orange Sherbet

Party Punch

Popcorn

Each child was given an apron and a chef's hat, which they later took home. (Instructions for making chef's hat and apron appear in Appendix G.) The children drew straws for partners and for the recipe they would prepare. I typed recipe sheets with step-by-step instructions for preparing sloppy joes, birthday cake, popcorn, and party punch. The sherbet had to be made in advance. I divided my kitchen into four areas. In each one I placed the necessary ingredients, utensils, and instructions for one recipe. A sign above the stove read: *Always wash your hands before you start to cook.* With clean hands and wearing their chef's attire the cooks proceeded with the preparation. They had a marvelous time, and since they had done the cooking, everything was absolutely delicious. I had planned to send any leftovers home with the guests, so their parents could share in their culinary feats. But there were none!

SLOPPY JOES

SERVES 8

(1 sloppy joe=3 meat exchanges, ½ vegetable exchange, 2½ fat exchanges, and 2 bread exchanges)

YOU WILL NEED

MEASURING CUP   CHOPPING BOARD   CHOPPING KNIFE

SAUCEPAN   MEASURING SPOONS   FRYING PAN

Shaker of salt
1 pound lean ground beef
½ cup chopped onion
1½ tablespoons butter
1½ tablespoons flour
1 cup tomato juice

1 tablespoon prepared mustard
½ teaspoon salt
Dash pepper
8 buns, split and toasted
8 ounces mild Cheddar cheese, shredded

1. Sprinkle bottom of frying pan lightly with salt from shaker.
2. Add ground beef and cook over low heat until browned.
3. Add onion and cook until tender.
4. Melt butter in saucepan over low heat.

5. Gradually add flour, stirring constantly.
6. Gradually add tomato juice, stirring constantly until smooth.
7. Add mustard, salt, and pepper and pour over meat. Cook over low heat for 10 minutes. Stir occasionally.
8. Serve on half of bun. Top with 1 ounce shredded cheese and remaining half of bun.

CARROT CURLS

(½ cup=1 vegetable exchange)

Cut a carrot in half lengthwise. Using a vegetable peeler, cut thin lengthwise strips from the flat side of the carrot. Roll each into a curl, secure with a toothpick, and crisp in ice water.

BIRTHDAY CAKE

Preheat oven to 350° F.   SERVES 8

(1 serving=1 bread exchange and 2 fat exchanges)

YOU WILL NEED

MEASURING CUP   MEASURING SPOONS   1-QUART PYREX DISH
                                                 OR LOAF PAN

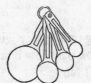
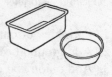

WOODEN SPOON   FLOUR SIFTER   WAXED PAPER

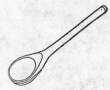

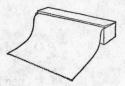

1½ cups sifted flour
5 teaspoons granulated sugar
    substitute (substitute for 1 cup
    sugar)
1 teaspoon baking soda
½ teaspoon salt

3 tablespoons cocoa
1 teaspoon vanilla
1 teaspoon vinegar
5 tablespoons melted butter or
    margarine, or vegetable oil
1 cup cold water

1. Preheat oven to 350° F.
2. Sift flour onto waxed paper and measure.
3. Mix flour, sweetener, baking soda, salt, and cocoa in an ungreased 1-quart Pyrex dish or loaf pan.
4. Make 3 holes in dry ingredients.
5. In first hole put vanilla; in second hole put vinegar; in third hole put melted butter.
6. Pour cold water over all. Mix until smooth.
7. Bake for 35 minutes.
8. Cool and frost in pan.

I don't recommend serving this cake at a dinner party for your gourmet friends. It does not rise very high and is best served right from the pan. But children love it, especially when they bake it themselves.

FROSTING FOR BIRTHDAY CAKE

(need not be counted as an exchange)

YOU WILL NEED

MEASURING CUP   WOODEN SPOON   SAUCEPAN

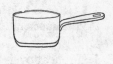

RUBBER SCRAPER

1-ounce package artificially sweetened low-calorie chocolate pudding
1 cup skim milk

1. Empty pudding into saucepan.
2. Gradually add milk. Stir over medium heat until mixture comes to a boil.
3. Remove from heat. Cool and frost cake with rubber scraper.

PARTY PUNCH

SERVES 8

(1 cup=1 fruit exchange)

YOU WILL NEED

MEASURING CUP   PUNCH BOWL   PARING KNIFE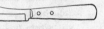

BOTTLE OPENER

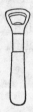

1 quart artificially sweetened cranberry juice, chilled

2 cups unsweetened pineapple juice, chilled

1½ cups lemon juice, chilled

2 oranges, sliced

2 10-ounce bottles artificially sweetened lemon-lime soda, chilled

3 tablespoons granulated sugar substitute (substitute for 2 cups sugar)

1. Combine all ingredients in the punch bowl.
2. Add several trays of ice.

ORANGE SHERBET

SERVES 8

(1 serving=⅓ fruit exchange)

1½ teaspoons plain gelatin
¾ cup water
¼ cup skim milk
¾ teaspoon granulated sugar
  substitute (substitute for 3
  tablespoons sugar)

1½ cups orange juice
1 teaspoon lemon juice
Pinch salt
2 egg whites, stiffly beaten

Dissolve gelatin in ¼ cup cold water. Bring ½ cup water to a boil. Add gelatin, milk, and sweetener. Mix well and remove from heat. Add orange juice, lemon juice, and salt. Pour into freezer tray and chill until mixture starts to thicken. Pour into chilled bowl and beat until mushy. Fold in egg whites. Return to freezer and chill until firm.

POPCORN

SERVES 8

(1 cup=⅓ bread exchange)

YOU WILL NEED

ELECTRIC POPCORN POPPER OR COVERED 3-QUART
SAUCEPAN

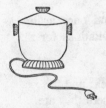

MEASURING SPOONS   MEASURING CUP   SERVING BOWL

  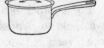

4 tablespoons cooking or vegetable oil (preferably corn oil)
⅔ cup popcorn
Salt to taste

1. Heat oil in saucepan.
2. Add popcorn.
3. Cover and shake until popcorn stops popping.
4. Remove from heat and pour into serving bowl.
5. Salt to taste.

OR

1. If an electric corn popper is used, pour oil into pan of popper.
2. Add popcorn.
3. Plug cord into electric outlet.
4. When rapid popping action begins to slow, pull cord from electric outlet.
5. As soon as popping has ceased, pull cord from base of popper, and pour into serving bowl.
6. Salt to taste.

Also included at the party were unsweetened pickles, which need not be counted as an exchange.

For another birthday we had a "Hobo Party" and once again I was able to bypass the traditional party sweets. Invitations for this event read as follows:

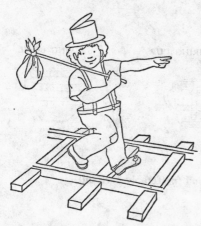

Hobos wander near and far,
Never certain where they are.
Some ride the rails,
Some hike the trails.
They live a life that's fun and
   free,
Come be a hobo for a day.
Arrive at noon on Saturday.
Be sure to wear the proper attire,
Prepared to hike and cook over a
   fire.
A prize will be given,
For the most appropriate
   apparel.

Refreshments were tied up in a red bandana attached to a stick. The children went off on a "Penny Hike,"† which culminated in a

---

† At every turn along the trail a coin is tossed. Heads means make a right turn; tails means make a left turn. Oh yes: Don't forget to send along an adult who knows the area.

picnic and a ride on a steam freight train, great fun, if one happens to be available. Once again Sherry helped to plan the menu:

Grilled Hamburgers
Celery and Carrot Sticks   Unsweetened Pickles
Cupcakes   Hand Fruit‡
Pink Lemonade

GRILLED HAMBURGERS

SERVES 8

(1 serving=2 meat exchanges, 1 fat exchange, and 2 bread exchanges)

1 pound ground beef	¼ cup dry bread crumbs
1 egg, slightly beaten	¼ cup minced onion
1½ teaspoons salt	8 hamburger buns, split and
¼ teaspoon pepper	toasted

Mix all ingredients and form into 8 patties. Place on grill 6 inches above glowing coals. Cook about 15 minutes, turning every 5 minutes.

CHOCOLATE CUPCAKES

Preheat oven to 350° F.   YIELDS 16 CUPCAKES

(1 cupcake=½ bread exchange and 1 fat exchange)

Use Birthday Cake* recipe. Spoon batter into paper-lined cupcake pans, filling about two-thirds full. Bake for 12 to 15 minutes. Cool and frost with Frosting for Birthday Cake*.

‡ See Appendix A, Fruit Exchanges.

PINK LEMONADE

SERVES 8

(1 serving=½ fruit exchange)

2 cups lemon juice
3 tablespoons granulated sugar
substitute (substitute for 2 cups
sugar)

5 cups water
½ cup artificially unsweetened
cranberry juice

Combine all ingredients. Pour over ice cubes from 1 tray. Additional sweetener may be added to suit individual taste.

The other contents of the bandana do not need recipes, but their exchange values are as follows: celery and carrot sticks: ½ cup=1 vegetable exchange; unsweetened pickles: "free food"; hand fruit: 1 small=1 fruit exchange.

As Sherry reached adolescence, the format for her parties changed, but eating was still the number one priority. Teenagers make their own plans and all I knew about the latest affair was when it would be held and that I was in charge of food. Her confidence in me was heartwarming. She didn't even ask about the menu.

I tried to use as many "free foods" as possible. I served quite a variety of unsweetened pickles along with:

Gazpacho
Raw Vegetable Platter   Horseradish Dip
Pickled Frankfurters
Party Pizza
Watermelon Bowl
Spicy Apple Cider

GAZPACHO

SERVES 12

(1 serving=1 vegetable exchange)

4 cups diced tomatoes
1½ cups chopped green pepper
¾ cup chopped onion
1 clove garlic, crushed
2 cups beef bouillon
½ cup lemon juice

1 tablespoon paprika
1 teaspoon salt
Freshly ground black pepper to
    taste
½ cup sliced cucumber

Combine all ingredients except cucumber. Let stand at room temperature for 1 hour. Chill for at least 2 hours. Serve garnished with cucumber slices.

RAW VEGETABLE PLATTER

(½ cup=1 vegetable exchange)

Asparagus: Serve raw tender spears 1½ inches long. Have them cold and crisp. Serve with a bowl of coarse salt for seasoning.

Broccoli and **cauliflower:** Break into bite-size flowerets and serve raw.

Carrot Curls*
Celery Curls*
Cherry tomatoes: Serve as is.
Cucumbers, peppers, summer squash, and **turnips.** Can be served cut in thin lengthwise sticks and crisped in cold water.
Radish roses: With a sharp knife, start at the root end and

make a cut between the red skin and the white flesh. Follow the curve of the radish almost to the stem. Crisp in ice water. Need not be counted as an exchange.

HORSERADISH DIP

(need not be counted as an exchange)

1 envelope low-calorie whipped topping	1½ teaspoons salt
½ cup water	4 teaspoons grated horseradish
2 teaspoons lemon juice	¼ teaspoon paprika

Beat whipped topping and water at high speed until thick and fluffy. Fold in remaining ingredients. Serve cold with tray of raw vegetables.

PICKLED FRANKFURTERS

SERVES 6

(3 frankfurters=1 meat exchange and 1 fat exchange)

Cover 1 pound cocktail frankfurters with boiling water and add:

¼ cup thinly sliced lemon	6 cloves
½ teaspoon peppercorns	1½ tablespoons salt

Cook until tender. Drain and pack in sterilized jars. Cover with:

1 cup white vinegar
¼ teaspoon granulated sugar substitute (substitute for 1 tablespoon sugar)
1 clove garlic

Refrigerate until ready to serve. Serve cold.

PARTY PIZZA

Preheat oven to 350° F.   SERVES 6

(1 serving=1 bread exchange, 1⅓ fat exchanges, 2 meat
exchanges, and 1 vegetable exchange)

2 6-ounce cans tomato paste	¼ pound salami
1 12-inch unbaked pizza shell	1 4-ounce can mushroom slices,
¼ pound boiled ham	drained
1 28-ounce can Italian plum	1 2-ounce can anchovy fillets,
tomatoes, drained	minced
¼ pound mozzarella cheese,	1 teaspoon oregano
thinly sliced	1 teaspoon basil
½ teaspoon salt	2 7¼-ounce cans pimiento
¼ teaspoon pepper	

Spread tomato paste over unbaked pizza shell. Spread ham over
tomato paste. Next place the drained tomatoes over the ham and
top with thin slices of mozzarella. Sprinkle with salt and pepper.
Top the cheese with salami, mushrooms, and anchovies. Sprinkle with oregano and basil. Cut whole pimientos in 4 places and
decorate the pizza by spreading them out in flowerlike arrange-
ments.

Bake for 20 minutes. Seasonings may be adjusted to suit individual taste.

WATERMELON BOWL

SERVES 12

(1 cup fruit=2 fruit exchanges)

Slice off the top of a well-shaped watermelon the long way.
Remove the watermelon meat and cut it into 1-inch cubes. Fill

the watermelon with cantaloupe balls, honeydew melon balls, fresh cubes of pineapple, the watermelon cubes, and thin slices of orange. Place the watermelon on a large serving platter and decorate it with clusters of grapes and long-stemmed cherries.

SPICY APPLE CIDER

SERVES 8

(½ cup=1½ fruit exchanges)

8 cups artificially sweetened apple juice
4 teaspoons grated orange peel

2 sticks cinnamon
10 whole cloves
2 oranges, sliced

Combine all ingredients. Bring to a boil. Reduce heat and simmer 5 minutes. Remove cinnamon and cloves. Serve hot or cold.

EASTER

And then came Easter! The greatest challenge of all. The traditional goodies in the Easter baskets were strictly off limits for Sherry. I didn't want to draw attention to her diabetic condition by making her treats any different from her brother's. As she was beyond the age of believing in the Easter Bunny, I couldn't pass the buck to that furry little creature. I was strictly on my own.

I diverted their attention from the customary candy by having a treasure hunt that sent them all over the house for nonedible surprises. It ultimately led to a miniature Easter basket for each filled with:

A Golden Rabbit‡
Decorated Hard-cooked Eggs
Peanut Butter Eggs   Coconut Cream Eggs

It was so much fun that it became an eagerly awaited annual event.

‡ See Appendix G.

HARD-COOKED EGGS

(1 egg=½ fat exchange and 1 meat exchange)

Simmer (do not boil) eggs for 15 to 20 minutes. Cool eggs by plunging them, at once, into cold water. To decorate, do your own thing.

PEANUT BUTTER EGGS

YIELDS 16 EGGS

(1 egg=1 fat exchange and ½ meat exchange)

1 cup peanut butter
3½ ounces nonfat dry milk
2½ teaspoons granulated sugar
  substitute (substitute for ½ cup
  sugar)

1 teaspoon sesame seeds (optional)
5 tablespoons water
Chocolate coating (below)

Combine all ingredients. Form into 16 eggs. Coat with chocolate coating, place on waxed paper, and refrigerate.

To simplify the coating process, insert a toothpick into the egg, then spread the coating on with a knife.

CHOCOLATE COATING

(need not be counted as an exchange)

6 tablespoons cocoa
2 tablespoons vegetable oil
2½ teaspoons granulated sugar substitute (substitute for ½ cup sugar)

Combine all ingredients and blend.

COCONUT CREAM EGGS

YIELDS 16 EGGS

(1 egg=¼ bread exchange and 1 fat exchange)

2 cups unseasoned mashed
  potatoes
1 tablespoon granulated sugar
  substitute (substitute for ½ cup
  plus 2 tablespoons sugar)

½ teaspoon vanilla
1 cup unsweetened shredded
  coconut
Chocolate coating (above)

Combine all ingredients and form into 16 eggs. Coat with chocolate coating, place on waxed paper, and refrigerate.

APPENDIXES

APPENDIX A

DAILY EXCHANGE WORK SHEET

The following chart is a daily exchange work sheet. Sheet One has sample menus that show you how easy it is to see at a glance what exchanges have been allotted and how many have been consumed. Sheet Two is a blank sample for your own use. The work sheet allows for flexibility in a given day and also allows for including snacks as part of the daily total.

	MILK		BREAD		MEAT		FAT		VEGETABLE		FRUIT	
BREAKFAST	½ cup skim milk		1 slice toast		1 soft-cooked egg		½ teaspoon butter 1 soft-cooked egg				1 cup orange juice	
	Allotment 1	Used ½	Allotment 2	Used 1	Allotment 1	Used 1	Allotment 1	Used 1	Allotment 0	Used 0	Allotment 2	Used 2
LUNCH	1 cup skim milk		1 hamburger bun		2 oz. lean ground beef		2 oz. lean ground beef		½ cup string beans			
	Allotment 1	Used 1	Allotment 1	Used 2	Allotment 2	Used 2	Allotment 1	Used 1	Allotment 1	Used 1	Allotment 1	Used 0
DINNER	½ cup skim milk		½ cup noodles		4 oz. tuna		1 teaspoon butter		½ cup broccoli ½ cup carrots		1 cup water packed fruit cocktail	
	Allotment ½	Used ½	Allotment 1	Used 1	Allotment 2	Used 2	Allotment 1	Used 1	Allotment 2	Used 2	Allotment 2	Used 2
SNACKS	½ cup skim milk										1 small apple	
		Used ½		Used 0		Used 0		Used 0		Used 0		Used 1
DAILY ALLOTMENT	2½		4		5		3		3		5	

	MILK		BREAD		MEAT		FAT		VEGETABLE		FRUIT	
BREAKFAST												
	Allotment	Used	Allotment	Used	Allotment	Used	Allotment	Used	Allotment	Used	Allotment	Used
LUNCH												
	Allotment	Used	Allotment	Used	Allotment	Used	Allotment	Used	Allotment	Used	Allotment	Used
DINNER												
	Allotment	Used	Allotment	Used	Allotment	Used	Allotment	Used	Allotment	Used	Allotment	Used
SNACKS												
		Used		Used		Used		Used		Used		Used

DAILY
ALLOTMENT

APPENDIX B

THE SIX EXCHANGES

(amount listed=1 exchange)

1. MILK EXCHANGES
Nonfat fortified milk

Skim or nonfat milk	1 cup
Powdered (nonfat dry, before adding liquid)	⅓ cup
Canned, evaporated skim milk	½ cup
Buttermilk made from skim milk	1 cup
Yogurt made from skim milk (plain, unflavored)	1 cup

Low-fat fortified milk

1% fat fortified milk (omit ½ fat exchange)	1 cup
2% fat fortified milk (omit 1 fat exchange)	1 cup
Yogurt made from 2% fortified milk (plain, unflavored) (omit 1 fat exchange)	1 cup

Whole milk (omit 2 fat exchanges)

Whole milk	1 cup
Canned, evaporated whole milk	½ cup
Buttermilk made from whole milk	1 cup
Yogurt made from whole milk (plain, unflavored)	1 cup

(½ cup=1 vegetable exchange)

2. VEGETABLE EXCHANGES

Asparagus	Greens:	Rhubarb
Bean sprouts	Beet	Rutabaga
Beets	Chards	Sauerkraut
Broccoli	Collards	String beans,
Brussels sprouts	Dandelion	green or yellow
Cabbage	Kale	Summer squash
Carrots	Mustard	Tomatoes
Cauliflower	Spinach	Tomato juice
Celery	Turnip	Turnips
Cucumbers	Mushrooms	Vegetable juice
Eggplant	Okra	cocktail
Green pepper	Onions	Zucchini

The following raw vegetables may be used as "free foods":

Chicory	Escarole	Radishes
Chinese cabbage	Lettuce	Watercress
Endive	Parsley	

Starchy vegetables are found on the Bread Exchange List.

(amount listed=1 exchange)

3. FRUIT EXCHANGES

Apple	1 small	Mango	½ small
Apple juice	⅓ cup	Melon	
Applesauce	½ cup	Cantaloupe	¼ small
(unsweetened)		Honeydew	⅛ medium
Apricots, fresh	2 medium	Watermelon	1 cup
Apricots, dried	4 halves	Nectarine	1 small
Banana	½ small	Orange	1 small
Berries		Orange juice	½ cup
Blackberries	½ cup	Papaya	¾ cup
Blueberries	½ cup	Peach	1 medium
Raspberries	½ cup	Pear	1 small
Strawberries	¾ cup	Persimmon, native	1 medium
Cherries	10 large	Pineapple	½ cup
Cider	⅓ cup	Pineapple juice	⅓ cup
Dates	2	Plums	2 medium
Fig, fresh	1	Prunes	2 medium
Fig, dried	1	Prune juice	¼ cup
Grapefruit	½	Raisins	2 tablespoons
Grapefruit juice	½ cup	Tangerine	1 medium
Grapes	12		
Grape juice	¼ cup		

Cranberries may be used as desired if no sugar is added.

Fruit may be used fresh or dried, canned or frozen, cooked or raw, as long as no sugar is added.

(amount listed=1 exchange)

4. BREAD EXCHANGES

Bread

White (including French and Italian)	1 slice
Whole wheat	1 slice
Rye or Pumpernickel	1 slice
Raisin	1 slice
Bagel, small	½
English muffin, small	½
Plain roll, bread	1
Frankfurter roll	½
Hamburger bun	½

Dried bread crumbs	3 tbsp.
Tortilla, 6″	1

Cereal

Bran flakes	½ cup
Other ready-to-eat unsweetened cereal	¾ cup
Puffed cereal (unfrosted)	1 cup
Cereal (cooked)	½ cup
Grits (cooked)	½ cup
Rice or barley (cooked)	½ cup
Pasta: spaghetti, noodles, macaroni (cooked)	½ cup
Popcorn (popped, no fat added)	3 cups
Cornmeal (dry)	2 tbsp.
Flour	2½ tbsp.
Wheat germ	¼ cup

Crackers

Arrowroot	3
Graham, 2½″ square	2
Matzo, 4″×6″	½
Oyster	20
Pretzels, 3⅛″ long×⅛″ diameter	25
Rye wafers, 2″×3½″	3
Saltines	6
Soda, 2½″ square	4

Dried Beans, peas, lentils

Beans, peas, lentils (dried and cooked)	½ cup
Baked Beans, no pork (canned)	¼ cup

Starchy Vegetables

Corn	⅓ cup
Corn on cob	1 small
Lima beans	½ cup
Parsnips	⅔ cup
Peas, green (canned or frozen)	½ cup
Potato, white	1 small
Potato (mashed)	½ cup
Pumpkin	¾ cup
Winter squash, acorn or butternut	½ cup
Yam or sweet potato	¼ cup

Prepared Foods

Biscuit, 2″ diameter	1
(omit 1 fat exchange)	
Corn Bread, 2″×2″×1″	1
(omit 1 fat exchange)	
Corn muffin, 2″ diameter	1
(omit 1 fat exchange)	
Crackers, round butter type	5
(omit 1 fat exchange)	
Muffin, plain, small	1
(omit 1 fat exchange)	
Potatoes, french fried, length 2″ to 3½″	8
(omit 1 fat exchange)	
Potato or corn chips	15
(omit 2 fat exchanges)	

Pancake, 5"×½"   1
   (omit 1 fat exchange)
Waffle, 5"×½"   1
   (omit 1 fat exchange)

(amount listed=1 exchange)

5. MEAT EXCHANGES

Lean Meat
Beef	baby beef (very lean), chipped beef, chuck, flank steak, tenderloin, plate ribs, plate skirt steak, round (bottom, top); all cuts rump, spare ribs, tripe	1 oz.
Lamb	leg, rib, sirloin, loin (roast and chops), shanks, shoulder	1 oz.
Pork	leg (whole rump, center shank), ham, smoked (center slices)	1 oz.
Veal	leg, loin, rib, shank, shoulder, cutlets	1 oz.
Poultry	meat without skin of chicken, turkey, Cornish hen, guinea hen, pheasant	1 oz.
Fish	any fresh or frozen	1 oz.
	canned salmon, tuna, mackerel, crab, lobster	¼ cup
	clams, oysters, scallops, shrimp	5 or 1 oz.
	sardines, drained	3
Cheese containing less than 5% butterfat		1 oz.
Cottage cheese, dry and 2% butterfat		¼ cup
Dried beans and peas (omit 1 bread exchange)		½ cup

Medium-Fat Meat: For each exchange of medium-fat meat
omit ½ fat exchange
Beef	ground (15% fat), corned beef (canned), rib eye, round (ground commercial)	1 oz.
Pork	loin (all cuts tenderloin), shoulder arm (picnic), shoulder blade, Boston butt, Canadian bacon, boiled ham	1 oz.
Liver, heart, kidney, and sweetbreads (these are high in cholesterol)		1 oz.
Cottage cheese, creamed		¼ cup
Cheese:	mozzarella, ricotta, farmer's cheese, Neufchâtel	1 oz.
	Parmesan	3 tbsp.
Egg (high in cholesterol)		1
Peanut Butter (omit 2 additional fat exchanges)		2 tbsp.

High-Fat Meat: For each exchange of high-fat meat
omit 1 fat exchange
Beef	brisket, corned beef brisket, ground beef (more than 20% fat), hamburger (commercial), chuck (ground commercial), roasts (rib), steaks (club and rib)	1 oz.
Lamb	breast	1 oz.

Pork	spare ribs, loin (back ribs), pork (ground), country-style ham, deviled ham	1 oz.
Veal	breast	1 oz.
Poultry	capon, duck (domestic), goose	1 oz.
Cheese	Cheddar types	1 oz.
Cold cuts		4½"×⅛" slice
Frankfurter		1 small

(amount listed=1 exchange)

6. FAT EXCHANGES

Margarine, soft, tub or stick†	1 tsp.
Avocado, 4" diameter‡	⅛
Oil: corn, cottonseed, safflower, soy, sunflower	1 tsp.
Oil, olive‡	1 tsp.
Oil, peanut‡	1 tsp.
Olives‡	5 small
Almonds‡	10 whole
Pecans‡	2 large whole
Peanuts, Spanish‡	20 whole
Peanuts, Virginia‡	10 whole
Walnuts	6 small
Nuts, other‡	6 small
Margarine, regular stick	1 tsp.
Butter	1 tsp.
Bacon fat	1 tsp.
Bacon, crisp	1 strip
Cream, light	2 tbsp.
Cream, sour	2 tbsp.
Cream, heavy	1 tbsp.
Cream cheese	1 tbsp.
French dressing§	1 tbsp.
Italian dressing§	1 tbsp.
Lard	1 tsp.
Mayonnaise§	1 tsp.
Salad dressing, mayonnaise type§	2 tsp.
Salt pork	¾" cube

† Made with corn, cottonseed, safflower, soy, or sunflower oil only.

‡ Fat content is primarily mono-unsaturated.

§ Can be used on fat-modified diet if made with corn, cottonseed, safflower, soy, or sunflower oil.

APPENDIX C

HERBS AND SPICES

Herbs: the leaves, seeds, or flowers of aromatic plants. Fresh herbs are preferable. Dried herbs should not be used in cold dishes. Use half as much of a dried herb as you would use of a fresh one.

Spices: the roots, bark, stems, buds, seeds, and fruit of aromatic tropical plants.

The following is a list of herbs and spices and their suggested uses:

Allspice	soups, broths, cucumbers, cabbage, beets, asparagus
Basil	fish, meat, artichokes, green beans, brussels sprouts, carrots, celery, corn, eggplant, onions, peas, spinach, all tomato dishes, broccoli
Bay leaf	soups, stews, pot roasts, tomato dishes, turnips, artichokes
Caraway	sauerkraut, soups, stew, green beans, brussels sprouts, broccoli
Cardamom	fruit compotes, turnips, asparagus
Chervil	soups, green salads, eggs, fish
Chives	green salads, eggs, fish, soups, tomatoes, squash, peas, corn, celery, cauliflower, green beans
Cinnamon	cooked fruits, puddings, squash, onions, red cabbage, beets
Clove	hams, carrots, beets, red cabbage, onions, tomatoes, turnips, squash, cauliflower
Curry powder	eggs, seafood, tomatoes, squash, eggplant, celery, broccoli, cauliflower, carrots, cabbage, green beans, artichokes
Dill	salads, fish, tomatoes, green beans, beets, broccoli, brussels sprouts, carrots, celery, cucumbers, onions, squash
Fennel	fish, chicken, spaghetti sauce, marinades, artichokes, cabbage
Ginger	meat, poultry, beets, carrots, leeks
Mace	fish, puddings, squash, cauliflower, carrots
Marjoram	poultry stuffing, meats, salads, all tomato dishes, green beans, carrots, cauliflower, squash
Mint	lamb, veal, cold drinks, fruits, frozen desserts, peas, carrots, green beans
Mustard	salad dressings, cheese dishes, asparagus, brussels sprouts, broccoli, celery, kohlrabi
Nutmeg	desserts, eggnog, spinach, squash, peas, onions, celery, cabbage, brussels sprouts, broccoli
Oregano	pizza, eggs, all tomato dishes, artichokes, green beans, broccoli, corn, peas, squash, eggplant
Paprika	fish, meat, poultry, onions, okra
Parsley	stuffings, soups, salads, meat and fish dishes, potatoes
Pepper	almost any food

Red pepper	seafood sauces, pizza, okra
Rosemary	lamb, beef, pork, broiled fish, boiled potatoes, green beans, asparagus, cauliflower, leeks, peas, squash
Saffron	rice, fish, stews
Sage	poultry and fish stuffings, pork, veal, carrots, eggplant, leeks, onions
Savory	poultry stuffing, meat loaf, peas, cauliflower, cabbage
Sesame seed	salads, noodles, rolls
Tarragon	eggs, poultry, fish, salads, peas, kohlrabi, cucumbers, celery, green beans, cabbage
Thyme	hamburgers, poultry stuffing, stews, green beans, beets, carrots, cauliflower, okra, leeks, onions, peas, squash

APPENDIX D

PEAK SEASONS FOR FRUITS

	Jan.	Feb.	Mar.	Apr.	May	Jun.	Jul.	Aug.	Sep.	Oct.	Nov.	Dec.
Apples	x	x	x	x	x	x	x	x	x	x	x	x
Avocados	x	x								x	x	x
Bananas	x	x	x	x	x	x	x	x	x	x	x	x
Berries						x	x	x				
Cantaloupe						x	x	x				
Cherries					x	x	x	x				
Cranberries	x	x								x	x	x
Grapefruit	x	x	x	x	x	x	x	x	x	x	x	x
Grapes	x	x	x	x	x	x	x	x	x	x	x	x
Honeydew								x	x			
Lemons	x	x	x	x	x	x	x	x	x	x	x	x
Melons					x	x	x	x	x	x		
Oranges	x	x	x	x	x	x	x	x	x	x	x	x
Peaches						x	x	x	x	x		
Pears	x	x	x	x	x	x	x	x	x	x	x	x
Persimmons										x	x	
Pineapples				x	x	x	x	x	x			

APPENDIX E

PEAK SEASONS FOR VEGETABLES

	Jan.	Feb.	Mar.	Apr.	May	Jun.	Jul.	Aug.	Sep.	Oct.	Nov.	Dec.
Artichokes		x	x	x							x	x
Asparagus			x	x								
Beets						x	x					
Brussels Sprouts	x	x	x					x	x	x	x	x
Cabbage	x	x	x	x	x							
Carrots					x	x	x					
Cauliflower	x	x	x	x								
Celery	x	x	x	x	x	x	x	x	x	x	x	x
Corn						x	x					
Cucumbers					x	x	x					
Eggplant							x	x	x			
Okra					x	x	x	x	x	x		
Green beans						x	x	x				
Parsnips	x	x	x									
Peas			x	x	x	x						
Scallions						x	x	x	x			
Spinach	x	x	x	x	x	x	x	x	x	x	x	x
Squash	x	x				x	x	x			x	x
Tomatoes							x	x	x	x		

APPENDIX F

EQUIVALENTS AND METRIC CONVERSION

1. EQUIVALENTS

1 dash or pinch	=less than ⅛ teaspoon
3 teaspoons	=1 tablespoon
4 tablespoons	=¼ cup
5⅓ tablespoons	=⅓ cup
12 tablespoons	=¾ cup
16 tablespoons	=1 cup
2 cups	=1 pint
2 pints	=1 quart
4 quarts	=1 gallon

1 teaspoon	=⅙ ounce
1 tablespoon	=½ ounce
2 tablespoons	=1 ounce
6⅔ tablespoons	=3½ ounces
1 cup	=8 ounces
1 pint	=16 ounces
1 quart	=32 ounces

Apples	—1 pound	=3½ cups, pared and sliced
Apricots	—1 pound	=3 cups dried, 6 cups cooked
Bananas	—1 pound	=2 cups, sliced
Beets	—1 pound	=2 cups, diced and cooked
Bread	—1 slice	=⅓ cup dry crumbs or 1 cup soft crumbs
Butter	—1 pound	=2 cups
Cabbage	—1 pound	=5 cups, shredded
Carrots	—1 pound	=2½ cups, sliced
Celery	—1 pound	=4 cups, diced
Cheese	—1 pound	=4 cups, grated
Chicken	—3½ pounds	=2 cups, cooked and diced
Cranberries	—1 pound	=4 cups
Garlic	—1 clove	=¼ teaspoon, chopped
Gelatin	—1 envelope	=1 tablespoon
Lemon	—1	=3 tablespoons juice
Lemon rind	—1	=3 teaspoons, grated
Lime	—1	=3 tablespoons juice
Meat	—1 pound	=2 cups, diced
Mushrooms	—½ pound	=2½ cups, sliced
Noodles	—1 cup	=2 cups, cooked
Onions	—1 medium	=½ cup, chopped

Orange	—1 medium	=⅓ cup juice
Orange rind	—1 medium	=2 teaspoons, grated
Peas in pod	—1 pound	=1 cup, shelled and cooked
Rice, raw	—1 cup	=3 cups, cooked
Rice, precooked	—1 cup	=2 cups, cooked
Shallots	—1 medium	=1 tablespoon, minced
Spaghetti	—1 pound	=7 cups, cooked

Tomatoes	—1 pound	=1½ cups, chopped
8-ounce can		=1 cup
10½-ounce can		=1¼ cups
12-ounce can		=1½ cups
No. 300 can		=1¾ cups
No. 303 can		=2 cups
No. 2 can		=2½ cups
No. 2½ can		=3½ cups
No. 10 can		=12–13 cups

2. METRIC CONVERSION

To change	to	Multiply by
Ounces	Grams	30.0
Pounds	Kilograms	0.45
Grams	Ounces	0.035
Kilograms	Pounds	2.2
Teaspoons	Milliliters	5.0
Tablespoons	Milliliters	15.0
Fluid ounces	Milliliters	30.0
Cups	Liters	0.24
Pints	Liters	0.47
Quarts	Liters	0.95
Gallons	Liters	3.8
Milliliters	Fluid ounces	0.03
Liters	Pints	2.1
Liters	Quarts	1.06
Liters	Gallons	0.26

APPENDIX G

CHEF'S HAT AND APRON

The chef's hat and apron are relatively easy to make. If you want to, you can make them more elaborate by adding trim or the guest's name.

The band of the chef's hat should be made from heavy white construction paper. Cut a strip 5″ wide and 20″ long from the construction paper (Fig. 1). Form a circle with the strip and staple or glue the ends together, overlapping about 1″ (Fig. 2).

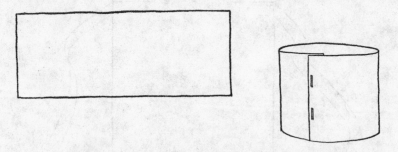

To make the upper part of the hat use white crepe paper. Cut a rectangular piece 22″ long and 10″ wide. Loosely roll your rectangle into a cone 20″ in diameter. Either sew, tape, or staple the overlapping ends together. About 1″ from the end of the cone gather the cone together and tie it up with either string or a "twist-em." Now turn the cone inside out, being careful not to tear it. Either staple or glue the inverted cone to the band. *Voilà*—one chef's hat! *Bon appétit.*

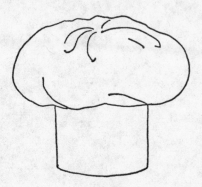

For the apron use a piece of muslin or an old sheet, preferably white. Cut a piece 22″ long by 18″ wide. About 18″ lengthwise, indent each side about 2″ to make the bib of the apron. Hem all sides of the apron. For the ties of the apron cut four pieces of material from the sheet, 12″ long and 1″ wide. Hem all ties and sew to sides and bib of apron.

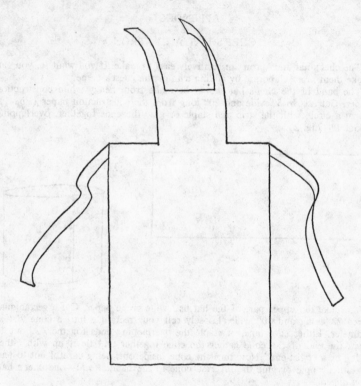

To make Golden Rabbits choose a large firm lemon for each rabbit. To make the long pointed ears, start about ½″ from top of lemon and outline ears with pencil or knife, drawing two lines for each ear about ¼″ apart at top and tapering to meet far down on the side. Cut just through peel to form ears. Carefully loosen and peel the ears upward and fasten in an erect position with a piece of wooden toothpick. With pin or toothpick, attach small puff of cotton at base of lemon for tail. On other side of lemon, cut out pieces of peel for eyes, nose, and mouth. Cloves, raisins, and cuts from colored gumdrops can be used to give expression to your Golden Rabbit's face.

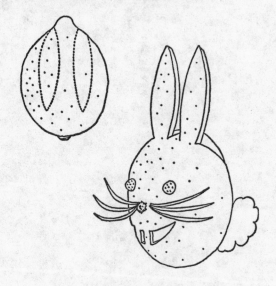

APPENDIX H

THE EXCHANGE SCOREBOARD

The purpose of the Exchange Scoreboard is to enable you to work with your child in computing the number of exchanges he consumes at times other than the meals that you prepare for him. If you will designate the foods that are permissible and the exchanges that they represent, your child can then transfer the information to the Exchange Scoreboard as he partakes of snacks in the course of each day. Every parent and child will work out his or her own system for this record keeping. However, it is important for your child to learn how to compute the exchanges, and it is important for you to know what he is eating, in order to balance his daily exchange intake.

I suggest you tape the Exchange Scoreboard to the door of your refrigerator, where it will be readily accessible to your child. Use decorative refrigerator door magnets (such as flowers, animals, etc.) to designate the exchanges consumed.

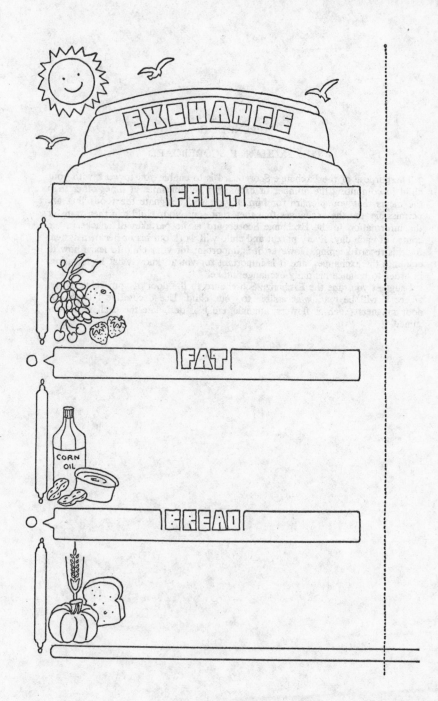

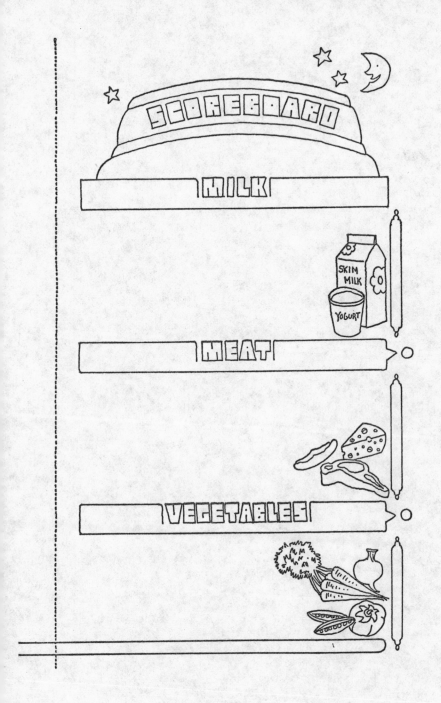

INDEX

American Diabetes Association, Inc.,
    4
Apple cheese potatoes, 90–91
Apple chips, 138
Apple cider, spicy, 29, 186
Apple grapefruit compote, 110
Apple juice, 29
    with beef broth, 29
Apple pancakes, 17
Apple Popsicles, 144–45
Apple rolls, 22, 30, 110–11
Apples, 30, 141
    baked, 109–10
Applesauce, 30, 111
    pork chops and, 58
Apple snow, 111–12
Apricot-raspberry soufflé, 122
Apricots, 141
Artichoke hearts, canned, in fruit
    salads, 103
Artichokes, with mock hollandaise,
    81–82
Artificial sweetener, 109
Asparagus
    buttered, 82–83
    raw, 183
Aspic, tomato, 101
Avocado, in fruit salads, 103

Baked apples, 109–10
Baked banana, 112
Baked beans, 163
Baked bean sandwich, 23
Baked custard, 30, 115
Baked ham, with orange glaze, 168
Banana and cottage cheese sandwich,
    23
Banana milk shake, 8, 128
Banana Popsicles, 145
Banana pudding, 30, 112–13
Bananas, 30, 141
    baked, 112
    and cranberry sauce, 114
Banana toast, 138
Barbecued chicken, 160
Barbecue sauce, 160–61
Basil, tomato slices with, 101–2
Beef, 43
    boiled, 46
    bourguignon, 47
    brisket, 46–47
    broiled fillet, 45

molded salad, 97–98
prime ribs, 44
roast fillet, 45
short ribs, 52
steak. *See* Beefsteak
stew, 28, 48
tongue, 54
Beef bouillon, 28
Beef broth, with apple juice, 29
Beef noodle casserole, 28, 75–76
Beefsteak
    broiled, 45
    fillet, 45
    flank, 48
    porterhouse, 45
    sirloin, 45
    Swiss, 53
    tenderloin, 45
Beef stew, 28, 48
Beets
    glazed, 84
    with horseradish, 83–84
Berries, fresh, 16
Beverages, 8, 127–35
    apple juice, 29
    banana milk shake, 8, 128
    breakfast, 8
    cocoa, 8, 29, 128
    commercial soft drinks, 127
    cranberry juice, 30
    diet soda, 127
    eggnog, 129
    free food, 127
    fruit juice, 8
    fruit punch, 130
    grapefruit juice, 30
    hot chocolate, 8, 130
    iced coffee, 130
    iced coffee cooler, 131
    iced tea, 162–63
    lemon punch, 131–32
    lime mist, 132
    nutrition snack, 132
    orangeade, 30, 133
    orange frost, 8, 133
    orange milk shake, 8, 30, 134
    party punch, 177
    pineapple fizz, 30
    pink lemonade, 22, 30, 182
    school lunch, 29, 30, 31
    spiced iced coffee, 131
    spiced tea, 134

U